# ARTHRITIS:
# The Doctors' Cure

# ARTHRITIS: The Doctors' Cure

Michael Loes, M.D., M.D.(H.)
Megan Shields, M.D.
Gary Wikholm, M.D.
David Steinman, M.A.

Foreword by
Gladys Taylor McGarey, M.D., M.D.(H.)

Keats Publishing, Inc.    New Canaan, Connecticut

*Arthritis: The Doctors' Cure* is not intended as medical advice. Its intent is solely informational and educational. The reader is encouraged to consult a qualified professional on specific personal health questions to insure that his or her situation has been evaluated carefully and that the choice of treatment is appropriate. The author and publisher expressly disclaim liability arising from the use or application of any information or treatments discussed in this book.

All patient names have been changed and certain identifying characteristics altered to protect their confidentiality and privacy.

**Library of Congress Cataloging-in-Publication Data**

Arthritis : the doctors' cure / Michael Loes,  . . . [et al.] ; foreword
   by Gladys Taylor McGarey.
        p.      cm.
   Includes bibliographical references and index.
   ISBN 0-87983-929-5
   1. Arthritis—Alternative treatment.    2. Glucosamine—Therapeutic
use.    I. Loes, Michael.
   RC933.A6654      1998
   616.7'2206—dc21                                              98-4273
                                                                   CIP

Printed in the United States of America

Keats Publishing, Inc.
27 Pine Street (Box 876)
New Canaan, Connecticut 06840-0876
Website address: www.keats.com

This book is dedicated to our patients who have persistently sought and searched out natural healing pathways without extensive reliance on medical drugs.

# Contents

# Acknowledgements

We would like to thank the following people for their assistance in reviewing or otherwise preparing this manuscript: Marliese Annefeld, Ph.D., for her extrmely helpful technical review of our manuscript; Michael Janson, M.D., for his perceptive review; Terry Zeyen for his excellent research assistance; Michael Murray, N.D., for his insightful writing on healing herbs and nutrients; Terry Lemerond of Enzymatic Therapy, for his usual high level of encouragement, enthusiasm and motivation; our editor Phyllis Herman for her artful editing of the manuscript; and Norman Goldfind of Keats Publishing, for his unflagging enthusiasm in seeing this project through.

# Foreword

I put on the cloak of a physician in 1946 in Ohio, first in Cincinnati and then in Wellsville, both on the banks of the Ohio River. The patients that were the most difficult for me to work with were those who were suffering from arthritis of various kinds. In the Ohio Valley with the high humidity summer and winter there were many, many people who were struggling with this problem. I felt terrible when I had to make the diagnosis early on for a patient, and particularly bad for patients who had suffered with it for long periods of time because I had no way of helping either. It was a progressive disease, associated with almost intolerable pain, frequently progressing to complete immobility. The lucky ones were in wheelchairs and the unlucky ones were immobilized in bed. As physicians, we want to relieve suffering and when we find ourselves in situations where there is so very little that we can do, it becomes the hardest part of our work.

In the 1940s and 1950s, the only things that we knew that would give patients some relief were liniments, heat, trying to keep them mobile, and aspirin. In our office we had three different colors of aspirin and frequently for a particular patient the pink aspirin wouldn't work, but the green would. For another patient the white aspirin worked better than the green. We knew that attitudes and emotions had something to do with the problem and a person's belief system certainly helped. But we had no validation of this either in our medical training or in the literature that was coming out at the time. Later on I began to notice that the patients who were willing to change their diets seemed to do better than those who wouldn't. The diet of most of the people in the Ohio Valley was meat, potatoes and gravy, topped with apple pie and ice cream. It seemed like the most common ways of fixing the meat and potatoes was by frying them. Lard and Crisco were the fats that were used, and margarine had just come into its own. People drank huge amounts of coffee with spoonfuls of sugar and cream. They drank water only on occasion. So, if I had to make the diagnosis of arthritis, I had little to offer the patient in the way of help.

When we moved out to Phoenix in 1955, it seemed a little better for people suffering from arthritis. The weather was better, the patients were beginning to look at diet a little differently, accepting whole grain bread rather than white bread, fruits were more available and vegetables and salads were more frequently used in the diet. Patients actually responded to cutting back on dairy, sugar, and red meats, and the medical literature actually began to change a little bit in that there were some comments about diet in association with various disease processes. The use of biofeedback was beginning to break through with the mind-body connection becoming more apparent.

Things have changed a great deal over this span of 50 years. Now when I have a patient who comes in, and I either make the diagnosis of arthritis or they come in with the diagnosis already made, my heart does not fall into my shoes. I look forward to working with them and watching them take control of their lives and begin to turn this disease around. As people take responsibility for their own health, which includes diet, exercise, massage, attitudes and emotions, the tables have really turned on arthritis. And now to be able to have some specific therapeutic agents, such as glucosamine sulfate available to use with patients and medical literature to back it up—this is truly a new era in medicine.

At the age of 77, and after having had multiple injuries to my right hip, I found myself two years ago in a great deal of pain, and had difficult walking, because of arthritis in the hip. Now with the use of the glucosamine sulfate and other therapeutic modalities I am almost completely pain free and walk without a limp and without a cane. So, it pleases me a great deal to see *Arthritis: The Doctors' Cure* published, which will give physicians tools to work with and give our patients a greater understanding of not only the disease process but how they can overcome it.

**Gladys Taylor McGarey, M.D., M.D.(H.)**

# Introduction:
## Not *Medicine as Usual*

## Who We Are

We are a group of physicians and educators who realize that
the usual methods for treating arthritis, especially osteoarthritis
and rheumatoid arthritis, are shortsighted. Typically, the healing
response is not enhanced and the drugs employed are, to be blunt,
all too often not only *not* in the patients' best interests, but
possibly damaging to their long-term health. The body deserves
healing nutrients, not just what an insurance company will pay
for or what a doctor, whose knowledge may be limited when it
comes to nutritional and other complementary strategies, chooses
to prescribe.

Above all, we consider ourselves educators, and we believe
that education is really what being a doctor is all about. Strictly
speaking, a doctor is a teacher. Teaching health is the best way to
help patients. As one expert notes, "Teaching safe and natural
healing methods is the most important missing piece in our North
American health care system."[1] We doctors perform at our
best—and in the true spirit of the ancient father of medicine,
Hippocrates—when we *teach* patients how to stay healthy.

We're extremely pleased to be part of the movement that is

bringing the complementary medicine message to doctors in the United States. It is our task as healers and educators to impart what wisdom we have accumulated, and to empower our patients and others in need of health counselling to create healthy independence and freedom from potentially dangerous treatments that may mask symptoms but do not stimulate the body's healing pathways.

> *We doctors perform at our best—and in the true spirit of the ancient father of medicine, Hippocrates—when we teach patients how to stay healthy.*

Our goal in this book is to help you unlock your body's own healing powers to rejuvenate your joints and provide greater mobility. Today's conventional painkiller approach to osteoarthritis is changing quickly and will soon be outdated. Our intention is to bring you information about all of the latest, safest and most effective breakthroughs for arthritis treatment. We also want to alert you to the exaggerated claims for certain drugs, nutritional supplements or other therapies which can be harmful—and costly.

We know that pain relief isn't going far enough. We must not simply mask symptoms but stop degeneration and rejuvenate the joints.

Many drugs are available to treat arthritis, yet only glucosamine sulfate is proven to relieve pain and stimulate joint regeneration. Moreover, it is completely safe. We will provide you a pathway for turning on the healing powers within your own body by using this nutritional supplement and by emphasizing a holistic approach encompassing diet, exercise, stretching, other nutrients and weight loss when necessary.

## The Difference Between Healing and Treatment

"What is the difference between *treatment* and *healing*? This is a key question for anyone who truly desires optimal health. Treatment, in the narrowest sense, involves drugs or surgery, utilizing some foreign substance, often alien to the body's natural ecology, to stop symptoms from the outside. Treatment does not address the root of the problem. Of course, certain emergencies, such as bacterial pneumonia or a broken leg, do require immediate *treatment* of some kind. Healing, on the other hand, stimulates the body's own natural powers, thus promoting a longer and healthier life. Deepak Chopra, M.D., physician and author, points out that one's body, when all is said and done, is the greatest healing pharmacy. Turning on the healing powers of one's own body is key to health.

# PART I

# 1
# True Stories of Real-life Healing

## *Sally*

Sally was a 45-year-old woman on half a dozen different medications for her arthritis. She had a high school education and came from a farming community in eastern Ventura County. She was seeking help from a medical doctor who knew about "herbs and things like that."

An examination revealed that she had very little flexibility remaining in her hands; her grip strength was weak. She said she hadn't been able to close her fist in years. Her wrists made a grinding noise and her fingers were disfigured by nodular prominences (known as Heberden nodes). What's more, magnetic resonance imaging (MRI) revealed that the cartilage in her hips had clearly eroded, making virtually all movement involving sitting, bending and twisting extremely painful and torturous. That wasn't all. She was distraught and withdrawn. She sat meekly in the exam room and with her hands drawn up against her body.

She was a pleasant woman, but seemed listless and numb with physical pain from long-standing arthritis. This was clearly a case where any physician would truly want to help, eager to counsel the patient on what she would need to do.

"It's this arthritis. Everything is painful. Doctor, please help!" More medication was not the answer. Her body's own healing processes needed to be restored.

Sally desperately needed help. The medically prescribed drugs she was on were more a random concoction than a regimen of effective medication and were causing increasingly troublesome side effects. The anti-inflammatory medications were ripping up her stomach like a bulldozer. She was suffering troubling fluid retention, increased blood pressure and diarrhea. She had a metallic taste in her mouth and had lost her desire to eat. She was tired and had bad headaches. She was also very depressed when her friends suggested she needed more medicine. They wanted her to use the popular mood elevators of the day, which she already knew had various other side effects. That was why she had come. Her life had turned into a toxic, poisonous morass.

This is the kind of case where a physician realizes that much of the responsibility for healing lies with the patient. Sally wanted to start healing, and that was the message that her body was crying out for her doctors to hear. Her own self-motivation would prove to be extremely important to her success. Any individual's self-motivation is, in fact, essential to regaining or maintaining health.

Prescription drugs were modern medicine's answer to Sally's woes, but what she needed most was to get back to health *basics* and turn on the healing powers of her own body.

Her new doctor, the one who knew about "herbs and things like that," began to talk to her in a completely different manner than any doctor had before, taking time to listen to her and really counsel her as an individual on what she needed to do. For the first time, Sally felt really comfortable with her doctor. He was using words like *healing* instead of *anti-inflammatory this* and *corticosteroid that*.

Sally's doctor designed a comprehensive healing program for

her. It would require time and commitment. It would certainly take weeks and probably months. It would be worth it though, because she could begin to reverse her arthritis and get back to her old (younger) self. The doctor told her he could tell her what to do, but she would have to take responsibility for her own healing. She would need to change her diet by getting off all junk food laced with hydrogenated and polyunsaturated oils and using olive, flaxseed and other safer and healthier oils and fats instead. She was to get back to a more ideal weight by sensibly increasing her activity and cutting back on calories, especially sugars, which are often eaten during times of stress or socializing instead of being eaten out of true need. He even suggested eating organically grown foods and markedly decreasing her consumption of red meat, pork and other fatty flesh foods. She was to begin a basic nutritional supplement program consisting of vitamins and minerals and other nutrients that would provide a solid nutritional foundation. These included nutrients with antioxidant fire power such as vitamins C and E, green tea and minerals such as magnesium, manganese, boron and selenium. In addition to these, it would be crucial to take glucosamine sulfate, 500 mg, three times per day.

The doctor sent Sally off, hoping that in two or three months time her own healing powers would be turned on. Yet, time and commitment would be needed. For Sally, it ultimately would lead to a new way of life.

She had to learn to make health her number-one priority. She had to use the motivation she possessed to begin healing herself with changes in diet, weight management and regular use of glucosamine sulfate.

The results were the reward. It took barely a month. Sally was clearly walking better as she reentered the doctor's office. She was lighter, better nourished and certainly happier. She was able to sign her name without having to painfully grip the pen.

She could get up and down from the exam table easily. Even her voice was stronger. On her three-month visit, she related that she was out picnicking with her family and played some soccer with her six-year-old granddaughter. Within a year, she had stopped using all medications—remaining only on her glucosamine sulfate program.

Sally's success story is not all that unusual for those who are already familiar with sensible nutritional supplements and the increasing knowledge that glucosamine sulfate works and works extremely well in cases of osteoarthritis. It is the kind of happy ending that we have learned to expect from many arthritis patients today. We'll tell you a lot more about glucosamine sulfate as we go along. For now, it was thrilling to hear Sally say, "I can walk. I can move without pain. I feel great!"

Let's analyze what happened here, because Sally is an actual case history. She had real problems; some mornings she would awaken wondering if death wouldn't be a more pleasing alternative to the aching in her joints and her constant hip pain. And Sally's case isn't unique. Many people today are questioning the purpose of living with such excruciating pain and loss of mobility. Thankfully, Sally is healed, but it took real seeking on her part, plus great discipline and a will to be healthy. Let this woman, without even a high school education, who spoke broken English, be an inspiration to all of us: We can heal our bodies ourselves, with the help of enlightened health professionals.

Western medical technology has made our diagnostic and emergency medicine skills the best in the world. In Sally's case, exotic technology was not needed, however. All the patient needed was some commonsense-guided medical advice and a supervised nutritional supplement program with glucosamine sulfate as required. She needed some information and a reasonable explanation for why she should take glucosamine sulfate and initiate the lifestyle changes that her doctor was advocating.

Nothing exotic. Just good, old-fashioned, patient-centered medicine by a physician who practiced integrative medicine at its best.

She definitely did not need more drugs.

We'll tell you more about the arthritis healing program that has worked for hundreds of our patients as we go on in this book, but for now let's enjoy the heartening news: *Arthritis can be healed.* There is help, but you must seek that help.

## Chet

A former high school varsity basketball player from New York, Chet prided himself on the fact that even in middle age he could go to the local high school and give youths half his age a good run for their money on the hard court. One day, Chet felt a twinge in his knee. The pain progressively worsened. Eventually, he found himself in his doctor's office seeking a prescription for painkillers. He said he had begun to give up hope of ever getting off painkillers or of ever dribbling down the basketball court again. He and his doctor talked. Fortunately for Chet, this doctor knew about healing strategies for arthritis sufferers.

Chet was defensive. He wasn't sure about "this alternative medicine stuff." He added he had a great health insurance policy. "I've been to the very best specialists. I know there's nothing that can be done except surgery, and I'm told that surgery doesn't always work. I've tried everything. I'm gaining weight and depressed. Worst of all, the word *old* finally has real meaning."

Stepping from the scale, Chet had a disturbed, dark look.

"Gosh, I weigh 220. Doc, I'm an elephant. You have any ideas?"

He told me about how it all started, the first twinges, the lack of cushion when he landed on the hardwood and rounds of painkillers. We placed Chet on an osteoarthritis healing program, including a commonsense diet that he could live with, daily stretching for 20 to 30 minutes and the use of glucosamine sulfate three times daily.

A month later, Chet's knees felt good enough for him to start dribbling at the school courts down the road from where he lived. Pretty soon he was taking a few practice shots.

Some guys came by. They were one short of a three-on-three and asked Chet if he wouldn't like to join them. Reluctantly, Chet started playing. "I don't know about this," he remembered saying to the guy. "I'm just an old guy!"

Amazingly, he felt light again, springy. When Chet went up for a rebound, he actually touched the rim. As he landed, he felt a renewed sence of cushioning in his joints and he realized his body was healing.

"Old?" he said later on in his doctor's office. "What do I know about old?"


*Laura*


Laura, a 46-year-old nurse practitioner who works in a ped-iatrician's office in Rhode Island, was suffering from aching joints. Ironically, so was her husband, Bob, who worked for United Parcel Service. It was a classic case of both partners in a marriage ultimately sharing the same ailment—osteoarthritis. In the office where she worked, Laura knew of a woman who was taking glucosamine sulfate. She called to discuss it and was encouraged by her report. Taking two grams a day, Laura and Bob found it put a lot more mobility and life back into their joints, relieving their pain and helping to restore the cushion and spring that helped them on their evening walks and allowed them to bicycle on the weekend. "Glucosamine sulfate really is joint food," she says. "It works!"

These cases represent only a few of the hundreds of case reports our team of doctors has collected from our patients who focus on healing from *within* rather than simply on treatment. Glucosamine sulfate truly is "joint food." It is a great discovery. It works. It is safe. It is practical and cost-effective.

## The Glucosamine Sulfate Story

As different as each of the above cases are, they have a lot in common with each other too: sensible diet; exercise and stretching; attention to lifestyle; use of select nutritional supplements and glucosamine sulfate spelled success, enabling each person to eventually be free from disabling immobility and joint pain.

Glucosamine sulfate is the substance used in multiple European studies where it was proven to be effective in the treatment of osteoarthritis. It has been accepted as a superior long-term strategy by the World Health Organization and was officially classified as a slow-acting drug in osteoarthritis by the International League Against Rheumatism.[2] More than 6,000 patients have been studied in some 20 clinical trials, both short-term and long-term. These studies have come to the same conclusion: glucosamine sulfate *works*. It should be forcefully noted that it is the "sulfate," not the chloride, acetylated, amide or chelate that has received stringent clinical testing. It is the purified glucosamine sulfate from Rotta Research Laboratories in Milano, Italy, whose glucosamine sulfate, extracted through a patented extraction method from ocean sea shell material, was used in these studies. Since glucosamine sulfate itself is not available to be patented, be aware that other extraction methods may not yield the same effectiveness. Classified as a nutritional supplement in the United States, supplemental forms of glucosamine sulfate can differ in many ways, such as in purity, fillers, compacting agents, delivery system and even the ratio of active to inactive constituents. This, in turn, affects absorption, distribution, binding, metabolic excretion pattern and ultimately the effectiveness of the product at the desired site in the body: the joints.

## Why Haven't I Heard About Glucosamine Sulfate?

Obviously and sadly, your doctor may not know about glucosamine sulfate. It is not trendy to accept European studies as the basis for clinical opinion. Historically, the primary bias may lay with the Food and Drug Administration (FDA) or arguably with our medical education system which tends not to teach nutrition or the use of vitamin and mineral therapies. Also, American medical journals rarely publish articles on nutrition. Most conventionally trained doctors feel more comfortable recommending pharmaceutical drugs.

The good news is that this is beginning to change. Not only are many of the European supplement and herbal companies exerting their financial clout with massive advertising campaigns in select media outlets, they are acting as global companies, advertising and selling by international routes and beginning multinational clinical trials. Only recently, *Arthritis Today*, published by the Arthritis Foundation, began to accept advertising for glucosamine sulfate. By reading this book, you, too, are on the cutting edge of modern medicine and healing. What's more, because our information systems are now global, you can search the European data banks as well as Medline by simply surfing the Internet. The information is there and the quality of the data is as good, if not better, than much of the research done in America.

In the pages that follow, we will present and discuss much of the available information on glucosamine sulfate. This discussion is not without controversy.

*The Arthritis Cure* by Jason Theodosakis, M.D. and co-authors is but one example of a popular book that recommends a combination of nutrients which have never been shown to be effective when used together in clinical trials. At least, no results of these clinical trials have been published in any European, American or other peer-reviewed scientific or medical journal (see also Chapter 6). Without being confrontative, our book offers additional data and a proven method to rebuild degenerative cartilage faster and more permanently, backed by studies on more than 6,000 patients.

## Other Arthritis Treatments

In preparation for this book, we reviewed the results of hundreds of clinical trials and other studies on many different arthritis treatments. We examined the medically prescribed and over-the-counter (OTC) drugs commonly used throughout America and Europe. We critically examined how glucosamine sulfate compared to these other commonly used medications. We were especially careful to look for studies in which glucosamine sulfate was compared to commonly used OTC drugs such as the non-steroidal anti-inflammatory class of drugs (NSAIDS), including ibuprofen and diclofenac. Utilizing our combined clinical experience spanning some 50 years in medicine, we reviewed more than 200 studies on the use of aspirin and other NSAIDs in the treatment of arthritis. We wanted to know what toxicity problems were most prevalent and what you, the consumer, really need to know regarding the use of these powerful OTC drugs which are part of the $7 billion pain-reliever industry—in America alone.

The NSAIDs, such as aspirin and ibuprofen, are beneficial in that they help to reduce swelling, heat and pain. However, even though the patient may feel better, no rebuilding of the cartilage occurs and further degeneration may actually occur. We found that while the most commonly recommended NSAIDs have some limited benefit in the short run, in the long run they simply cannot match glucosamine sulfate for either efficacy or safety.

*The NSAIDs, such as aspirin and ibuprofen, are beneficial and help to reduce swelling, heat and pain. The patient may feel better, but no rebuilding of the cartilage occurs and further degeneration may actually occur. We found while the most commonly recommended NSAIDs have some limited benefit in the short run, in the long run they simply cannot match glucosamine sulfate for either efficacy or safety.*

On the other hand we agree that antioxidants have a theoretical and clinical basis for their effectiveness in either preventing or slowing down overall degenerative processes including for various forms of arthritis. We believe that the free radical theory of aging, using antioxidant nutrients such as vitamins, minerals and herbs, is an extremely important part of disease prevention and turning on the healing process within. The use of antioxidants will someday be recognized as one of the most significant contributions to the health of the 20th century. It's clear that you also need basic vitamins and minerals, which often function as antioxidants and as building blocks for structural support. What's more, antioxidants play an important role in fighting off the damaging effects of inflammation by quenching the devastating microcellular effects of free radicals that exert so much cumulative damage on joint tissues. However, it is also clear that you need glucosamine sulfate to rebuild the joints, and you probably do *not* need chondroitin sulfate.

There are also substances, such as the NSAIDs, that reduce inflammation in the short run but may prevent normal rebuilding processes necessary to continue an active life. The NSAIDs are beneficial in that they are anti-inflammatories; they stop or slow down inflammation. Hence, they reduce redness, swelling, heat and pain. They probably make the patient feel better quickly, but they do have common side effects. What's more, these agents do not rebuild cartilage. They do not enhance the healing response, either; in fact, they probably retard the healing process. Unlike glucosamine sulfate, they are not classified as slow-acting arthritis drugs by the International League Against Rheumatism nor do they have the safety profile of glucosamine.

Complementary (alternative) strategies for controlling the pain of arthritis and reversing arthritis-related degeneration of cartilage such as acupuncture, homeopathy and clinical hypnosis also have extensive literature and experience to support their use in the right patient population and in the treatment hands of experienced practitioners in these disciplines. To comprehensively discuss these therapeutic strategies, however, is beyond the scope of this book; some sources of information on holistic and alternative medicine are listed in the Resource section in the back of the book.

# The Benefits of Glucosamine Sulfate

It is our opinion that glucosamine sulfate offers the first long-term osteoarthritis treatment option with proven healing and safety. This is especially true when compared to corticosteroids and less potent anti-inflammatories. It is not our intent to disparage other claims, and we recognize the occasional specific need for these latter agents, but for mainstream prevention and reversal, glucosamine sulfate makes more sense and costs less. The toxic effects of the NSAIDs and corticosteroids are well-known, particularly, upset stomach (epigastritis), kidney disease (interstitial nephritis) and liver damage (hepatocellular mitochondrial damage). We present information not only as physicians, but as consumer advocates, hoping that your healing path will be a quick journey that doesn't waste precious time or valuable dollars on unproved therapies. We feel that this book is especially important because it comes at a time when pharmaceutical companies, according to *The Wall Street Journal,* are likely to be launching heavy advertising campaigns for arthritis prescription drugs on television and other forms of mass media.[3] They hope that consumers will ask their physicians for these drugs because they saw them on TV. In a mass-media campaign, it is unlikely that the risks will receive as much time and space as the benefits of these therapies. It is imperative that consumers be informed. Health knowledge is more important today than ever. By being informed, you are actually helping doctors to do their job better as well as protecting your health.

In spite of all the research, many doctors will continue to remain skeptical that a natural substance like glucosamine sulfate works. They will continue to argue that glucosamine sulfate has no scientific evidence because they will not accept findings from the European clinical trials. It is very interesting that reliable knowledge stops just east of New York, according to the FDA.

Harris McIlwain and Debra Fulghum Bruce, authors of *Stop Osteoarthritis Now!,* state, in regard to glucosamine sulfate, "Unfortunately, there has been no specific evidence that these supplements help patients with osteoarthritis."[4] They are wrong. They are clearly not familiar with the extensive data accumulated in European trials. We believe it is our task to reach mainstream doctors with this important information.

## How This Book Can Help You

You can turn on the amazing healing powers in your own body and initiate dramatic improvements in your health if you are suffering from rheumatoid arthritis, osteoarthritis, or one of the many other forms of arthritis by following our comprehensive 10-point program. It consists of the following elements:

- Proper diet.
- Food elimination, if necessary.
- Daily use of glucosamine sulfate.
- Use of additional secondary arthritis-healing nutrients and other holistic health strategies.
- Aerobic and conditioning exercise plus stretching.
- Weight loss, if necessary.
- Avoidance of repetitive motion.
- Use of biomechanics and ergonomics.
- Stress reduction.
- A positive outlook on life—even in the face of adverse circumstances such as painful joints.

Osteoarthritis is the most common joint disease, and frequently likened to a rusty hinge that needs to be warmed up by a hot shower in the morning. Yet other forms of arthritis are common, particularly rheumatoid arthritis. All of these forms of arthritis will respond to the 10-point comprehensive healing program discussed here. Yet, we emphasize again that you should work with your doctor. We are doctors and health educators, and recognize that sometimes potent complex pharmacotherapy will be necessary to stop an acute flare-up and prevent joint destruction. Nonetheless, as noted in the case histories of Sally, Chet and

Laura, most of what we see is the common presentation of progressive cartilage loss, increased weight-dependent pain and progressive loss of function and well-being. Our program can stop this. This book will tell you how to reverse much, and hopefully all, of this. We're here to coax, persuade and motivate you to get your life back on track by committing to our 10-point healing program.

---

10 Steps to Pain-Free Joints

Arthritis is America's number-one crippler, affecting an estimated 40 million patients, including 80 percent of people over the age of 50. Throughout our professional careers, we've discovered that joint health is a common concern for many people. Whether you're one of the four out of five baby boomers who wants to prevent osteoarthritis, or who is simply interested in improving joint function, here are our ten simple steps to help alleviate pain and insure healthier joint structure:

1. *Practice good nutrition*. Stay away from fatty foods that consist mainly of sugars, starches and refined carbohydrates—all of which can worsen arthritis. A vegetarian diet is often helpful, but not essential. Keeping off the extra pounds keeps further stress off joints.

2. *Try a selective elimination diet.* Under a physician's supervision, eliminating some foods occasionally may also stop a food trigger that could be aggravating your osteoarthritis.

3. *Use glucosamine sulfate daily.* The nutritional supplement glucosamine sulfate has been medically proven to help to rebuild cartilage. We

recommend using a stabilized form available in many health food stores.

4. ***Take supplements.*** Vitamins and minerals are important additions to the diet.

5. ***Exercise regularly.*** Use it or lose it! Exercise is one of the most powerful tools available to you. If you suffer from osteoarthritis, aerobic activities such as walking, stretching and swimming can help strengthen muscles and bones to compensate for weakened joints.

6. ***Lose weight.*** Maintaining a healthy weight is essential. Overweight stresses the joints, causing the wear and tear that can lead to osteoarthritis.

7. ***Avoid repetitive motion altogether.*** Take breaks if your job or other activities involve repetitive motion. Stay away from repetitive-motion sports, such as tennis and golf.

8. ***Use biomechanics and ergonomics.*** Be aware of how you walk and sit; don't hunch your shoulders or slouch. Protect your joints when lifting or pulling by using carts or other devices equipped with wheels. Be sure your chair provides your shoulders and neck with the proper support.

9. ***Alleviate stress.*** Stress is part of life, but we can all learn to cope effectively. Take deep breaths or count to 10. A positive support group of family and friends is also helpful. Set aside time each day for the things that you enjoy. It'll help you to maintain a positive outlook.

10. ***Keep the right attitude.*** Take time every day to visualize how your life will be improved when your physical and mental health are at their best.

# 2
## The Bionic Body

You complain of a twinge in the knee. You go to the doctor, who tells you to lie on the table. The doctor moves your leg in various ways and it hurts. You cry out when you get a twinge, a snap, a grind or a pop at the joint surface. Either conventional radiographs are ordered or magnetic resonance imaging (MRI) which hones in on the problem as a narrowed joint and a rough, cartilaginous surface. These reveal narrowing of the joints between the knee bones. That means your cartilage is worn down. Hopefully, there is still enough cartilage left to help cushion your bones during the day's jarring activities. In some patients, the cartilage has completely disappeared. You're diagnosed with osteoarthritis, and, if you're not careful from now on, you could eventually require extensive orthopedic surgery due to complete loss of your cartilage. You ask yourself: Why has this happened to *me*? Your doctor tells you it's from the "wear and tear" of daily living. The joints just wear out. In particular, your cartilage is becoming thin and dry and is starting to lose its cushioning effect. It's usually not too serious, your doctor goes on to explain. If you just stop doing jarring types of activity, you should be okay—for a while. Sure, you're thinking to yourself: "No more basketball, tennis or skiing. I'm too young for a sedentary life."

Your doctor goes on optimistically about all of the break-throughs that medical technology has developed for the replacement of natural joints with artificial ones. He tells you how artificial joints can be made from a combination of metal and plastic or porcelain. Successful joint replacement surgery, he explains, can improve movement and relieve pain. Although most commonly it's hips and knee joints that are replaced, he mentions that it is not at all uncommon anymore to perform joint replacement surgery for the ankles, shoulders, elbows and finger joints. Indeed, your doctor explains, he is one of the new school of physicians who has a great deal of faith in joint replacement surgery. Like many doctors today, he is more willing than ever to operate on younger patients and at an earlier stage in the disease. Of course, he explains, such surgery should only be undertaken when other treatments have failed to work. He goes on to mention that surgical replacement of your joints should last a good 10 to 15 years before you will need a second surgery to replace the worn-out parts. Yet he never mentions glucosamine sulfate. It is baffling that he does not talk about one of the few treatments that could actually help you to avoid the need for surgery altogether.

You leave the office, and your knees are hurting a little more. Maybe he's right, you say silently to yourself. Maybe he's not, you hope. Sure, there is modern bionics, but how will you get through the security machine at the airport? Somehow you don't really laugh.

Sounds pretty bleak!

## Looking for Alternatives

It is time to search for options. What if you could avoid surgery altogether? Who wants to be a bionic man or woman, anyway? Knowing that lifestyle changes such as diet and exercise plus targeted nutritional supplements and herbs can help is the empowering first step.

### WHAT DO I TELL MY DOCTOR
### IF I WANT TO START TO USE GLUCOSAMINE SULFATE?

Glucosamine sulfate is completely safe. Because it so safe and without any drug interactions whatsoever, many people use glucosamine sulfate without medical advice from their doctor or other health professional. In many cases, this is acceptable. Some people, however, may find it more beneficial to work with their doctor or other health professional who can act as their "coach" and who can help them to design a specific, comprehensive healing program. What's more, your informed health care advisor can help you measure your healing progress with objective benchmarks by measuring improvements in mobility and freedom from pain quantitatively.

If you are on a medical drug or involved in any medical procedures or have any possible health concerns, it is always best to talk with a trusted, qualified health care professional when designing a supplement program. Having said this, some doctors may be open and some not to your using glucosamine sulfate. If your doctor is reluctant to recommend it, you may wish to locate a doctor who will be of more help to you. Check the Resources section in the back of this book to find the names of organizations who can provide you with doctors in your area who are familiar with the use of this supplement. In addition, we have established an information center to provide pertinent glucosamine sulfate literature for doctors and other health care professionals. (see Resources)

Show your doctor this book, if necessary. We have endeavored to present solid, factual information aimed at the mainstream medical community, particularly medical consumers and their care givers.

# 3
# Fire in the Joints

Health is mobility. If you don't have mobility, you don't have health. It's really that simple. Imagine that your joints are like a "rusty door hinge," creaking, sticking and just not moving. This is what happens with arthritis. Some people liken the pain of arthritis to a fire in the joints, burning, inflaming their tissues. Others use words like "gritty," "grinding" and "popping" to describe the condition of their inflamed joints. No matter how individuals describe their individual case of arthritis, the fact is that this condition is painful and debilitating. It is a robber of joy and happiness and one that is becoming increasingly prevalent among the American population, especially among the aging baby boomer generation.

Imagine the following images either now or perhaps when you are older—and in your 50s, 60s, or beyond . . . Imagine . . .

- *Being at a party with a lively band, yet not being able to dance;*
- *Sitting at home on a glorious fall evening unable to take an evening walk;*
- *Not being able to hike up to your favorite vista or mountain peak to see the clouds blowing in over the mountains or the ocean or prairie lands spread below.*

- *Pounding pain from the concrete that you walk on—as if your legs and feet are drumming;*
- *Reaching for a package of scotch tape or another small item, at your home or at the store but being unable to actually grip it or even open a package because your hands and fingers are so inflamed that they have lost their flexibility and strength.*

These images are real. This is what happens with arthritis. These are images to which we can all relate. They reflect everyday actions that we take for granted. What's more, such problems, like those that we've described, happen far more often than you might think. However, thanks to supplemental nutrients and other health strategies, we may finally be able to do something so that these limitations will not be as common in the future as they are today.

Yes, health is mobility, and our loss of mobility affects our mental, as well as physical, well-being.

We are all likely to experience some form of arthritis as we grow older. It has been estimated that as many as four out of five of the 80 million baby boomers in America today will eventually begin to lose mobility, the first sign of arthritis. Fortunately, we can now do something to protect our bodies from crippling arthritis.


## What is Arthritis?

The 19th century London physicist Sir Archibald Gerrod described and named this widespread crippler that today we call arthritis.

Arthritis, literally translated, means "fire in the joints." In its simplest definition, arthritis is an inflammatory disease of the joints. Although more than 100 different forms of the disease have been identified in the field of rheumatology (the scientific name for the study of arthritis), two types are most prevalent: osteoarthritis and rheumatoid arthritis. Generally speaking, we can divide the types of arthritis into two larger categories: inflammatory, immune-related arthritis and simple or mechanical osteoarthritis.

*Arthritis comes in more than 100 varieties. Most forms of this disease include some joint degeneration as part of their pathology. That is why a substance such as glucosamine sulfate, which actually rebuilds the joints, is so important.*

### THE FIVE MOST COMMON FORMS OF ARTHRITIS

**Rheumatoid arthritis:** An inflammatory and immune-mediated disease, rheumatoid arthritis, also known simply as RA, is estimated to affect up to 10 million people—usually women.

**Ankylosing spondylitis (spinal arthritis):** Causing immobility of the back, and often the shoulders and neck, ankylosing spondylitis, an inflammatory form of arthritis, affects more than 300,000 people—usually men.

**Gout:** Usually associated with lifestyle and diet, gout affects some one million persons—usually men.

**Osteoarthritis:** The most common form of arthritis, osteoarthritis, affects from 15 to 20 million Americans— usually over age 45. Far more people are likely to be afflicted with osteoarthritis than rheumatoid arthritis. Whereas osteoarthritis tends to damage larger weigh-bearing joints, rheumatoid arthritis attacks the body's smaller joints, such as the fingers and wrists, usually symmetrically. Both forms of the disease can be crippling to the sufferer.

**Systemic Lupus Erythematosus (SLE):** Technically not an arthritis but an immune-related form of arthralgia often affecting the large and small joints, SLE affects about 131,000 people—usually women.

## Rheumatoid Arthritis

Rheumatoid arthritis is a chronic disease of the joints characterized by alternating periods of active inflammation and absence of symptoms, both of variable duration. Some of the symptoms include a sense of utter fatigue and weakness, plus a very slight fever. The joints may become just a little stiff at first, but a few weeks later they become much stiffer and swollen. The stiffness and swelling may start in the small joints, such as the fingers and wrists, but progress to larger joints and afflict both the joints and bodily organs. This is a total body disease, affecting the body inside and outside. Interestingly, symmetrical joints, such as the hands, wrists and ankles, are often hit first with an attack. The joints may even be "hot" to the touch. About one-third of rheumatoid arthritis patients are luckier than most, and only one or two joint areas are affected; for most, the pain is spread throughout the entire body.

About eight to ten million Americans have rheumatoid arthritis. The usual age at which it strikes is in the 20 to 40 age group. In terms of gender differentiation, rheumatoid arthritis is most likely to strike women aged 36 to 50, according to the National Rheumatism Foundation. The next major target is men 45 to 60. Some children and teenagers suffer various forms of rheumatoid arthritis.

Ordinarily, the immune system repels threats to health from bacteria, viruses and chemical toxins, as well as diseased, damaged cells and other types of pathogens. Thankfully, our immune system's powerful yet complex army of defenders—the B-cells, T-cells, antibodies and macrophages (debris eaters)—generally devour, digest and otherwise disarm external threats to our health.

In rheumatoid arthritis, however, the immune system is out of control and turns on the body. Although medical science is unsure of the exact cause of rheumatoid arthritis, we do know that the body's immune system begins to form antibodies, then circulating immune complexes that cause a chronic inflammation of the joints. An antibody is a group of protein molecules produced as a primary immune defense by the immune system's lymphocytes; it is the B-cells that produce antibodies that attack and defuse foreign substances in the body; each antibody has a uniquely shaped site that combines with a foreign substance such as a virus or toxin and disables it. Eventually, however, these antibodies combine with antigens and other cellular fragments to form large immune complexes that become deposited in joint tissues and are so misshapen and foreign to the body itself that they themselves are attacked by the immune system, setting off a cascade of inflammatory events. Thus, the immune system begins attacking itself, resulting in inflammation and joint destruction.

In rheumatoid arthritis, it is the thin membrane surrounding the joints (synovium) that becomes swollen and extremely inflamed. As attacks continue to occur, the bones and joint tissues are weakened, eventually destroying the integrity of the joint, including the cartilage which provides a cushioning effect. This battle within the immune system is likely to spread beyond the borders of the joints and throughout the body, damaging and killing off the red blood cells, which then leads to a constellation of symptoms within the body, including weakness, fatigue and swelling.

The formation of these new antibodies may be heightened due to a variety of influences on a person's health. One's genes, for example, may make one vulnerable to foreign toxins, food allergies and biological pathogens such as bacteria and viruses, which can initiate an immune firestorm. However, other influences under our direct control, including lifestyle and diet, can potentiate the firestorm, as can allergies. We can subdue this unwelcome immune whirlpool of activity and inflammation by ingesting the safest foods and supplements, many of which will be discussed in Part III.

Small joints are usually most affected, including finger and toe joints. Yet, the wrists, knees, ankles and the small interlocking joints of the neck can also be targeted. However, less known is that this inflammation can spread to the eyes, heart, lungs and blood vessels.

Some experts believe that rheumatoid arthritis can be caused by allergens, especially those in the diet, combined with a permeable intestinal wall (leaky gut syndrome). James Braly, M.D., medical director of Immuno Labs, Inc., of Fort Lauderdale, Florida, notes:

> Five to ten years ago, it would have been heresy to state that allergens could induce arthritis and that, by the elimination of those allergens, the arthritis would go into remission. Now it's accepted among most rheumatologists and allergists that some people do have allergy-induced arthritis. A primary cause of most rheumatoid arthritis appears to be delayed food allergy and the often related problem of abnormal permeability of the intestinal wall.[5]

According to this theory, partially digested food particles pass through the intestinal wall into the bloodstream. These unintentional "invaders" are then deposited in the body's joint and other tissues, where they can cause an inflammatory response as the body's immune system mobilizes to disarm them.

It is not as well-known, but bacterial infections may be at the root of some cases of rheumatoid arthritis. Other microbial invaders, including protozoa, yeast and fungus, can also cause or aggravate arthritis. Finally, some medical drugs, such as diuretes, may trigger arthritis. And for some, albeit a small percentage, arthritis may simply be genetic.

Rheumatoid arthritis has a very subtle method of attack. You might not even realize that your body is under attack. In the *Family Medical Guide,* the American Medical Association expertly describes the disease's onset:

Rheumatoid arthritis may begin without obvious symptoms in the joints. Over several weeks or even months you may feel generally ill, listless and without appetite. You are likely to lose weight and to have vague muscular pains and possibly a low-grade fever. Only later do you develop the joint symptoms that are typically characteristic of rheumatoid arthritis. In other cases, the inflammation flares up suddenly, without previous symptoms of any kind. When your joints are affected, they become red, warm, swollen, tender to the touch, painful to move and stiff. The stiffness is usually most noticeable first thing in the morning. As you move and exercise the joints, the pain and stiffness gradually become less severe.[6]

Although rheumatoid arthritis is a complex disease whose causes are not extremely well understood, help is available. Glucosamine sulfate may be helpful for certain aspects of rheumatoid arthritis, particularly for helping to maintain cartilage in as healthy a state as possible, and two other supplements—fish

oils and combination enzymes in particular—offer further promise for rheumatoid arthritis sufferers (see Chapter 9).

Other nutrients, such as zinc and thymus gland extract, may be
able to help to re-educate the body's immune system as well as
decrease gut permeability and other risk factors for rheumatoid
arthritis.

Diagnosis of rheumatoid arthritis may be based on physical
symptoms, such as whole body aching, weakness, fatigue and
swollen joints that are usually symmetrically afflicted. If the
disease has progressed farther, joint deformities may have
already occurred. The terms used to describe these deformities
include swan neck, *boutonnière* and cock-up toes (also called
hammertoe).

One's blood profile can also offer telltale signs of the onset of
rheumatoid arthritis. A number of blood diagnostic tests can point
to the RA diagnosis.

- **Sedimentation Rate.** High sedimentation rates indicate
  active inflammation.
- **Anemia.** Very low levels of hemoglobin in the red blood
  cells.
- **Immune system dysfunction.** The blood contains immuno-
  globulins or immune complexes which, with the onset of
  rheumatoid arthritis, become so altered that the body produces new antibodies to zap these altered immune proteins.

X-rays and MRIs, can reveal swelling, cartilage degradation
and narrowing between joints, all of which occur as the cartilage
disappears.

## *Ankylosing Spondylitis*

Ankylosing spondylitis is a severe inflammatory arthritis of unknown cause. Its association with the gene linkage called HLA-B27 strongly indicates that genetic factors are important in the expression of the disease. Evidence suggests that the disease occurs when a genetically predisposed person comes into contact with certain bacteria (*Klebsiella* being a candidate), viruses and environmental factors, not yet identified.

This form of arthritis will make life miserable with severe back pain, often moving into the middle and upper back area all the way up to the neck, sometimes to the point where movement in any direction is severely limited; for the sufferer, even turning the head, bending or stooping may be difficult, if not nearly impossible to do without great pain. It is as if one's spinal column is fused into place. Early morning stiffness and many other physical limitations accompany this condition. In its advanced form, almost total immobilization of the spine, called the straight "poker spine," may result.

At first, the sufferer may feel that he simply has a strained back. However, instead of getting better, his condition worsens. Mornings, when the sufferer arises from bed, can be particularly troubling, with spinal pain that lasts for hours. Over time, the pain becomes greater, mobility is more limited and the suffering can be extremely painful.

This very troubling condition affects some 300,000 people and is especially common in men.

Medical science is not sure about the causes of ankylosing spondylitis. One plausible theory attributes its onset to a tissue condition. As we mentioned people with it have tissues with a gene linkage known as HLA-B27 that closely mimic in appearance a bacteria called *Klebsiella*, which usually resides in the bowel, feeds on starchy carbohydrates and multiplies. The body produces antibodies that destroy healthy tissues that look like this bacteria including HLA-B27 cells in your tissues. The end result is the deposition of fibrous tissues. This leads to stiff, painful, immobile joints and spine. See Chapter 7 for dietary tips for improving this condition.

Activity and pain relievers are probably the best antidote to this painful, all too often debilitating condition. If the condition becomes severe, the sufferer's posture may become deformed.

While ankylosing spondylitis is most likely immunologically mediated and genetically driven, this doesn't mean that it has to ravage one's joints. Stopping the inflammation and immunodys-regulation may require corticosteroids and potent immunological drugs to get on top of the destruction; rebuilding and preventing further downward spiraling is likely to involve antioxidant therapy.

About half of the people with this form of inflammatory arthritis also suffer from arthritis of the hips and shoulders. Also, in some cases, the disease actually may burn out after a few years, disappearing as mysteriously as it first appeared.

## Gout

As with ankylosing spondylitis, gout primarily affects men over the age of 40. About one million people suffer from gout. It also is another form of inflammatory arthritis, usually first appearing in the first metatarsal joint of the great toe. It is accompanied by pain, swelling and inflammation of the joint, making walking and standing extremely painful. The inflamed area is usually reddish-purple, shiny and dried out. Inside the joint are uric acid crystals which can be aspirated (painfully) to confirm the diagnosis. Other common sites where gout either first shows up or advances to are the joints of the hands, wrists, elbows, shoulders, ankles and knees. In fact, gout can even show up in the earlobes, causing what is called tophi (bumps), or tophaceous deposits, which are more amorphous globs of cellular debris encased with uric acid crystals. Not only are the joints sore with gout, but even the skin gets sensitive—so sensitive, in fact, that many gout sufferers cannot even tolerate a bed sheet over their painful joints. Other somewhat common sites of first occurrence include the hand, elbow or knee.

A metabolic accumulation of uric acid is both the cause and accelerator of gout. Various reasons may cause it to flare up such as lifestyle and environmental factors including alcohol, dehydration from excessive heat, smoking, or more direct causes such as taking diuretics, or after chemotherapy, when cellular destruction by prescribed toxic agents causes the level of uric acid to rise. When the kidney gets overloaded by the high levels of uric acid, the blood levels go up and uric acid starts entering the tissues and joints. Not only is further kidney damage caused, but stones may be formed and then further pain results.

Your doctor can help assess your risk of developing gout and treat it if it occurs. Gout, like other forms of arthritis, causes joint destruction. Strategies for preventing and healing gout are described in Chapters 7 and 9. It is very important, however, to work with a professional.

If left uncontrolled, gout can cause kidney disease, high blood pressure and joint deformity.

*Aspirin Warning*. Avoid aspirin if you're suffering from gout. Aspirin can actually slow the body's excretion of uric acid.

Another condition similar to gout is known as *pseudogout*. In this case, the cause is *not* uric acid. The villain is calcium pyrophosphate that it gets into and around the cartilage of the joint, causing it own brand of havoc. Pseudogout can mimic gout, presenting all of the same symptoms. Don't let the name mislead you. Pseudogout is not a less painful a condition.

## Infectious Arthritis

Almost any bacterium or fungi can cause arthritis, provided a route of penetration is available and the host (the patient) has a friendly terrain which isn't going to fight off the intruder. Bacterial infection of the joint—also known as infectious arthritis—is more common than is usually believed.[7]

Apart from the classical gonococcal arthritis (related to *Neisseria gonorrhea,* the same bacterium that causes gonorrhea), at least two types of arthritis are well known to be caused by infections. In particular, Lyme arthritis or Lyme disease and staph or staphylococcal arthritis are both caused by infectious organisms and may be successfully treated with antibiotics.

Weakening of the host's immune competence, preexisting joint damage and invasive diagnostic therapeutic procedures are the main risk factors for bacterial arthritis. The diagnosis can be suspected clinically, but must be confirmed by culture of the synovial fluid. Sometimes, a tissue biospy of the synovium is necessary to actually identify the specific bacteria causing infectious arthritis. Bone scanning, also known as scintigraphy, will help pick up local activity in a joint, making it look hot on the scan. While this test is helpful, it does not identify the organism or fungi causing the problem, which is the crucial information on which treatment is based.

Amplification of bacterial DNA by a technique known as polymerase chain reaction, which helps to produce many copies of the same bacterial gene, is a new procedure that could become an important tool for quick and accurate diagnosis.

Treatment is based on joint drainage and antibiotics, which

should be started as soon as the diagnosis is suspected. Additional strategies under investigation include the use of laboratory-produced monoclonal antibodies and substances that can modulate production of synovial fluid cytokines which cause inflammatory reactions.


## Osteoarthritis

Another name for osteoarthritis, *arthrosis*, literally means "degenerative joint disease." This certainly characterizes osteoarthritis, which usually becomes more apparent in older people, especially in the larger, weight-bearing joints, including the hips, knees and spine.

Under the age of 45, osteoarthritis is more common in men. However, after age 45 it is ten times more common in women than men.[8] Forty million Americans have some form of osteoarthritis, from mild to severe, including 80 percent of people over age 50. Some 20 million Americans suffer from disabling osteoarthritis. This number is likely to increase by three or four times over the next several decades. Also, people in specific types of occupations may be more affected than others, such as ballet dancers who get it in their feet after years of standing on their toes and football players after repeated trauma and injuries to the joints that occur during games.[9]

However, many of these people can be helped with lifestyle changes and glucosamine sulfate.

In osteoarthritis, the smooth lining of a joint, known as the articular cartilage, begins to flake and crack. With the loss of this protective cartilage, the underlying bone becomes thickened and distorted. Eventually, this may lead to episodes of pain, swelling and stiffness in the affected joint. These episodes may be chronic or occur at intervals of months or years. Some people may not even notice the swelling, while in other cases, affected joints may become extremely knobby and enlarged. Sometimes the pain seems to move from the affected joint to other areas of the body. This is known as referred pain. As one team of experts notes, "Osteoarthritis of the hip is sometimes felt most painfully in the front of the thigh and knee."[9]

What are the symptoms of osteoarthritis? Morning stiffness is one of the first. Pain after prolonged use of a certain joint is an early sign. The pain becomes worse with prolonged activity, better with rest. Loss of range of motion is another. The disturbing sense that your joints have crackled is a symptom that indicates the disease is worsening (crepitus). This is most likely to occur in the hips or knees. However, as the condition progresses, people may experience more pain—even without motion.

Many doctors say osteoarthritis is inevitable given the daily wear and tear on the body's joints. This just isn't true. We can make conditions much tougher for our joints by our personal lifestyle habits. Due to our increasingly inactive lifestyles and fatty diets, our joints are being asked to carry far more weight than ever before. Too many of us are junk food and television addicts. The joints just can't hold up to obesity and eventually do wear out. One-third of Americans are obese. Exercise and diet combined with weight loss are key, as is regular use of a quality glucosamine sulfate supplement.

## Arthritis-related Disorders

*Polymyalgia Rheumatica.* This disorder is not technically an arthritis but causes arthralgia—pain in the joint, but not true destruction. Commonly afflicting people over 50, polymyalgia rheumatica usually occurs in the area of the shoulders and hips, presenting severe nighttime and morning pain. Other affected areas of the body include the shoulders, arms, hips and thighs. Women are twice as likely as men to be afflicted with this fairly common disorder. This can be a bad news disease, causing inflammation in the arteries, anemia and enlarged spleen. It often requires low-dose steroids to keep it in control.

As with many cases of arthritis, OTC anti-inflammatory drugs and painkillers are often recommended for sufferers. Sometimes, however, more powerful corticosteroid drugs are prescribed; these may offer tremendous help. After a few years, polymyaglia rheumatica usually disappears with or without treatment.

*Systemic Lupus Erythematosus (SLE or Lupus).* As with polymyaglia rheumatica, SLE or lupus most often strikes women. However, unlike polymyaglia rheumatica, SLE strikes young women most often between the ages of 20 to 40. The condition is characterized by severe fatigue and butterfly rash across the face; debilitating pain and swelling often occur in the hands, wrists, elbows, knees, ankles or feet. There may also be morning stiffness in the joints. Other signs and symptoms of lupus include a worsening of the butterfly rash across the face following sun exposure, a pale or blue tinge to the fingers when exposed to cold and possibly hair loss.

Lupus is a serious condition because it may also cause diseases of the internal organs, including the heart, brain, lungs and kidneys, as well as bleeding, anemia and chronic infections. With proper treatment, however, lupus can be controlled, and sufferers can expect normal life expectancy.

Diagnosing lupus is not always easy. While some 95 percent of patients with lupus will have a positive test for antinuclear antibody (+ANA), which is an abnormal blood protein, approximately 5 to 10 percent of older patients will have this antibody in the absence of lupus. What is needed to make the diagnosis is a finding of the "rimmed pattern" of the ANA and a positive anti-double-stranded DNA test, which indicates that the cell's nucleic acids have been altered in response to the disease. To complete the diagnosis, if renal disease is present, one must have a kidney biopsy. Once the diagnosis is made, treatment is available. While lupus is usually not a primary cartilage destroying disease, patients with lupus are often put on high dose steroids for long periods of time causing their joints wear out sooner than they would without intake of steroids. Hence, the need for nutritional supplements, including antioxidant therapy. See Chapter 9.

## Arthritis: the Causes

**Living longer.** People are living longer than ever before. With age, the body's cartilage cells become worn and less efficient, resulting in scraping and grinding of bone on bone.

**Fatty diet, inactivity.** Obesity is a prime cause of osteoarthritis. The body's connective tissues can handle only so much weight before it is too much, and then they become strained to the point of breakage and deterioration.

**Nutritional Deficiencies.** The body becomes less able to digest foods as it ages and may not derive adequate nutrition from diet alone. Deficiencies of key vitamins, minerals and cartilage cell building-block nutrients can lead to increased risk for osteoarthritis by impairing the body's rebuilding processes.

**Allergens in the diet.** Sometimes allergens cause rheumatoid arthritis. Some people have problems with various meats, cheese or nitrite preservatives used to maintain the fresh look of cured meat and fish.

**Trauma.** Blunt force trauma is a prime cause of osteoarthritis, especially in athletes. Altogether too many professional football players have left the game with crippling osteoarthritis due to their bruising profession. High school and college athletes, especially those involved in football and other bruising contact sports, may also be susceptible to latent trauma effects.

**Repetitive movement.** Something as mild and yet repetitive as clicking a computer mouse all day can cause tightness and cracking in the shoulder and neck area, which may result in osteoarthritis. At the other extreme, working with a chain saw damages not only the cartilage of the arms and shoulders, but other joints as well. Another common cause is found in delivery workers who are constantly bending and lifting. Be wary of occupationally related osteoarthritis, which may result from repetitive movements or from placing too much pressure on specific joints in the body, such as the knees and hips.

**Poor biomechanics.** Walking and posture—the biomechanics of gait and posture—can be another cause of wear and tear on the joints and resulting osteoarthritis.

**Genetics.** In a small number of cases susceptibility to arthritis is inherited. It is estimated that six million Americans have arthritis susceptibility genes and are more likely to be afflicted.

Fortunately, in each of these cases, a comprehensive health program can help to tip the odds in favor of healing.

FIVE ARTHRITIS MYTHS

1. *You'll get osteoarthritis if you live long enough.*
   False. Osteoarthritis is *not* inevitable. By improving your diet, exercising and using nutritional supplements, you can dramatically reduce your risk of ever suffering a debilitating joint disease.

2. *There's nothing you can do about arthritis once you have it.*

   False. Changes in diet and lifestyle, together with intelligent use of nutritional supplements, can provide help to a great many arthritis sufferers, whether they are suffering from osteoarthritis or rheumatoid arthritis. In addition, glucosamine sulfate is safe, natural and proven to work for both relieving pain and rebuilding cartilage in a significant number of patients.

3. *Pharmaceutical painkillers relieve pain without side effects.*

   False. Evidence suggests that painkillers are likely to be used in higher and higher doses over time and cause long-term damage to the cartilage and bones by altering the body's cartilage cells' metabolism and reproduction. What's more, most OTC painkillers pose chronic toxicity problems to the kidneys and liver and they virtually all cause micro-bleeding in the gastrointestinal tract.

4. *Only people who've had traumatic injuries or who work in professions like professional football get osteoarthritis.*

   False. For example, a concert pianist, who spends his days hunched over his keyboard, may suffer forms of osteoarthritis. Ballet dancers are also known to suffer higher than normal rates of osteoarthritis. Anyone can get arthritis.

5. *If I have osteoarthritis, I will have to give up an active life.*

   False. In fact, most people with osteoarthritis can go on to live relatively, if not fully, active lives. Exercise, when done intelligently, is a healing elixir for the joints. Exercise forces fluids to be exchanged, moving nutrients in, debris and toxins out. Furthermore, modern medical technologies, if absolutely necessary, such as hip or knee replacement, can return lost mobility to arthritis sufferers.

# 4

# The Conventional Medical Treatment of Arthritis

We face a real dilemma as physicians. First, patients want quick pain relief. They come to the doctor's office and demand prescriptions they hope are going to be the magic bullet. Even though doctors know about the side effects of pharmaceutical drugs, particularly the very serious complications associated with the use of corticosteroids, we continue to prescribe these medications, hoping that the complications will be minimal and, yet provide much needed pain relief. Very often, physicians simply don't know about other safer avenues of treatment such as glucosamine sulfate.

Our job, as doctors, is to relieve pain. One in six Americans lives in pain. "No single sickness comes close to equaling pain in terms of the number of people affected," say Mary E. O'Brien, M.D. and Donna Hoel in a recent issue of *Postgraduate Medicine*.[10] Interestingly, they also observe, "Until recently, pain management, especially chronic pain management, was seldom included in medical curricula. In fact, pain was, and still generally is, considered an essential part of the human experience. Those who bear the greatest pain are accorded the greatest respect, and courage and moral strength continue to be tied up in the ability to withstand pain."

Pain is an important arthritis issue, but not the *sole* issue. Relieving pain should not be confused with rebuilding and regenerating joint tissues.

## Nonsteroidal Anti-inflammatory Drugs

Osteoarthritis today is usually treated with nonsteroidal anti-inflammatory drugs (NSAIDs) or analgesics. Examples of NSAIDs are aspirin, diclofenac and ibuprofen, which are quickly effective against pain and relieve the most disturbing symptoms for patients (see table 4.1). Other drugs, known as analgesics, are also used for pain relief, including acetaminophen (Tylenol), which has only weak anti-inflammatory properties and is not considered a true NSAID but is effective as an analgesic for mild to moderate pain. Almost all NSAIDs are orally administered, with the exception of ketorolac (Toradol), which is available both in oral and parenteral doses. Indomethacin and aspirin are available as suppositories. Only choline magnesium (Trilisate) comes in a liquid.

NSAIDs are an important component in balanced analgesia in the management of both acute and chronic pain. NSAIDs have a direct action on spinal nociceptive processing, with a relative order of potency which correlates with their capacity to inhibit the enzyme cyclo-oxygenase (also known as COX) activity. There are two metabolic forms of cyclo-oxygenase—COX-1 and COX-2. What's important to our discussion is that various NSAIDs inhibit the isoforms differently, and it is felt that when the COX-1/COX-2 inhibitory ratio is high, there are fewer gastric or kidney problems. For example, ketololac, nabumetone and the newer agent meloxicam appear to have far more favorable safety profiles than some older drugs such as piroxicam or tolmetin.

There are now nearly 30 pharmaceutical agents classified as NSAIDs (Table 4.1). There are also some nonsteroidal agents which have anti-inflammatory effects yet are not usually considered traditional NSAIDs. One is colchicine, which is largely effective only in acute gouty arthritis. It is not an analgesic and usually does not provide relief in other types of pain, though there is considerable evidence that this agent helps when administered intravenously in low back pain syndromes. Other agents which have anti-inflammatory effects but are not thought of as nonsteroidals are methotrexate, chloroquine, penicillamine and the gold salts. The major mechanism for these agents is immunological; and although they do have anti-inflammatory properties, these drugs are not generally discussed in the same context as NSAIDs.

One reason there are so many different brands of NSAIDs is that each particular drug works a little differently with individual patients. Each of the NSAIDs has varying chemical structures, and some authors have put them into different classes. Their metabolism, absorption, volume of distribution, protein-binding and elimination pathways in the body all vary according to their structure. What's more, there are drug interactions and effects on the blood which will also differ according to their structure. For example, indomethacin is a methylated indole, and sulindac, though closely related to indomethacin, is a sulfoxide. The side effects are very different. Indomethacin tends to cause fluid retention and headaches; sulindac does not. Indomethacin is, however, somehow effective in the headache syndrome known as *hemicrania continua*, and sulindac is not. Some doctors advocate that if one agent doesn't work, one should be selected from another class on the retrial. This view may not be well supported, at least as far as efficacy is concerned. If there are problematic side effects, however, then switching classes may be of some value.

TABLE 4.1

NONSTEROIDAL ANTI-INFLAMMATORY DRUGS (NSAIDs)
MOST COMMONLY USED FOR ARTHRITIS

| Generic Name | Trade Name | Usual Daily Dose |
|---|---|---|
| Aspirin | Bayer | 4-10g |
| Aspirin (12 hour) | Zorprin | 4-10g |
| Choline magnesium trisalicylate | Trilisate | 750 mg 2x |
| Diclofenac | Cataflam, Voltaren | 50 mg 2x |
| Diclofenate potassium | | 50 mg 3x |
| Diflunisal | Dolobid | 500 mg 2x |
| Etodolac | Dolobid, Lodine | 400 mg 3x |
| Fenoprofen | Nalfon | 600 mg 2x |
| Flurbiprofen | Ansaid | 100 mg 3x |
| Ibuprofen | Advil, Motrin, Nuprin | 800 mg 3x |
| Indomethacin | Indocin | 50 mg 3x |
| Ketoprofen | Orudis | 75 mg 3x |
| Ketoprofen delayed release | Oruvail | 200 mg 3x |
| Meclofenamate | Meclomen | 50 mg 3x |
| Mefanamic acid | Ponstel | 250 mg 4x |
| Nabumetone | Relafen | 1,000 mg 2x |
| Naproxen | Aleve, Anaprox | 500 mg 2x |
| Naproxyn | Naprosyn | 500 mg 2x |
| Oxyprozin | Daypro | 1,200 mg 4x |
| Piroxicam | Feldene | 20 mg 4x |
| Salsalate | Disalcid, Salfex, Mono-Gesic | 1,000 mg 2x |
| Sulindac | Clinoril | 200 mg 2x |
| Tolmetin | Tolectin | 400 mg 3x |

Most analgesics and NSAIDs, whether prescribed or purchased as OTC products off the drugstore shelf, can be safely used for two to three days. Obviously, instances occur when the use of these drugs is the best course of action, particularly for instances of acute pain. No one is calling into question their value in appropriate situations. However, in the case of arthritis, using these drugs long-term is a mistake because these drugs are simply anti-inflammatories. Unlike glucosamine sulfate, they do not stimulate healing.

TABLE 4.2

COMPARATIVE NSAID TOXICITY SCORES

| Drug | Toxicity Score<br>*from least toxic (1.00) to most toxic (9.00)* |
|------|------|
| Salsalate | 1.00 |
| Ibuprofen | 1.25 |
| Diclofenac | 3.57 |
| Fenoprofen | 3.57 |
| Sulindac | 4.75 |
| Naproxen | 5.20 |
| Ketoprofen | 6.00 |
| Indomethacin | 6.25 |
| Piroxicam | 8.00 |
| Tolmetin | 8.73 |
| Meclofenamate | 9.00 |

Data based on serious reactions per million prescriptions, based on data from the Committee on Safety of Medicine, *British Medical Journal*; 1986; 292: 614 and 292: 1190–1192, 1986; Griffin, M.R., et al. *Annals of Internal Medicine*, 1991; 114: 257–263; Fries, et al., *Arthritis, Rheumatology*, 1991; 34: 1353–1360.

Moreover, when these drugs are used for longer periods, virtually all patients suffer some complications which can range from microbleeding in the gastrointestinal tract to liver or kidney toxicity. It is extremely important when using these medications to follow all label instructions and precautions. (See Table 4.2 for a listing of the least to the most toxic NSAIDs.)

What's more, these medications may have interactions with other drugs. For this reason, those using other drugs, should use NSAIDs only if they have consulted with their physician. Also note, that smokers, people over 65, those with ulcers, and especially people on cortisone-type medications may all be advised not to take NSAIDs because of the greater risk for complications.

ARTHRITIS DRUG INTERACTIONS

**Antacids**—May decrease the absorption of NSAIDs.

**Anticoagulants**—As a group, NSAIDs are highly protein-bound and when given with anticoagulants such as coumadin, some displacement of coumadin into the blood will occur, hence potentiating the effect of coumadin. NSAIDs also inhibit platelet aggregation. The effect will parallel the drug elimination time. Hence, for drugs with long elimination times, such as piroxicam and oxyprozin, the effect will last for days. Giving NSAIDs to patients who are receiving blood thinning medication is not always contraindicated, but caution is advised. Because nonacetylated NSAIDs, such as salsalate and choline magnesium salicylate, do not directly effect platelet function, they may be safer but can still potentiate coumadin by displacing a protein-bound drug.

**Antirheumatic agents**—Many drugs used in rheumatoid arthritis, such as azothiaprin (Immuran), penacillamine (Depen, Cuprimine), gold compounds and methotrexate, cause bone marrow toxicity, including decreases in the white blood cells and platelets. NSAIDs may potentiate their toxicity.

**Corticosteroids**—Patients who take corticosteroids concurrently are at higher risk for NSAID-induced gastrointestinal diseases, including bleeding and ulcers.

**Diuretics**—The action of diuretics may be potentiated with concurrent use of NSAIDs.

**Lithium**—The pharmacologic activity of lithium is heightened in patients taking NSAIDs. One proposed mechanism is decreased kidney efficiency because of imbalances in the body's production of certain messenger chemicals called prostaglandins that affect kidney function.

**Oral hypoglycemia agents**—Several NSAIDs (fenoprofen, naproxen and piroxicam) have been noted to potentiate oral hypoglycemic agents.

**Phenytoin (Dilantin)**—The effect of phenytoin may be potentiated, again because NSAIDs have a high affinity for protein-binding sites and can displace it. This effect has been shown with the same agents noted to interact with oral hypoglycemic agents (fenoprofen, naproxen and piroxicam).

**Probenecid (Benemid)**—This agent has been shown to increase plasma levels of indomethacin, naproxen, ketoprofen and meclofenamate. Hence, a lower dosage of these NSAIDs is advised when given with probenecid.

Adapted from Hence, P.K. and Willkens, R.F. *Patient Care* (Review), December 15, 1994.

What about aspirin? One of the most commonly used OTC drugs is aspirin, which is commonly recommended for arthritis. It does, in fact, relieve pain and inflammation, it is inexpensive, and can also help to prevent heart attacks and strokes. But to ease arthritis pain, it often must be used at a very high dose, four to ten grams per day. At these doses, toxicity often occurs, most often tinnitus and gastric irritation. If using this pain reliever at all, it probably is better to use enterically coated aspirin. Better yet, we suggest glucosamine sulfate to address osteoarthritis-related problems, possibly in combination with an enzyme preparation that can also help to reduce inflammation. Persons with gout should never use aspirin because it can cause the body to retain uric acid.

## NSAIDs and Internal Bleeding

*The PDR Family Guide to Prescription Drugs* contains the following warning about ibuprofen (Advil or Motrin), indomethacin (Indocin), sulindac (Clinoril) and tolmetin sodium (Tolectin): "You should have frequent checkups with your doctor if you take ibuprofen [indocin, clinoril or tolectin] regularly. Ulcers or internal bleeding can occur without warning."[11]

In fact, this warning applies to virtually all NSAIDs. Because irritation to the stomach lining is so commonly associated with this broad family of drugs, some doctors may recommend that you also take misoprostol (Cytotec), a prostaglandin E1 look-alike which protects the stomach lining and decreases stomach acid. It is prescribed at 200 mcg four times a day with food and has been effective in decreasing gastric ulcers (not duodenal ulcers) in patients on NSAIDs. Although most of misoprostol's side effects (nausea, flatulence, headaches, dyspepsia, vomiting, constipation) are not life-threatening, the drug may cause miscarriage. Thus, it should never be given to women who are pregnant or who intend to become pregnant. The *Physicians' Desk Reference* gives it a black box warning, which is not to be taken lightly.

Although antacids and sucrafate (Carafate) are often given to patients complaining of hyperacidity, these agents have *not* been shown to decrease the incidence of gastric ulcers for patients on NSAIDs.

J.F. Fries and colleagues at Stanford have studied in patients with rheumatoid arthritis the problem of gastric complications over the past ten years by coordinating information from the American Rheumatism Association Medical Multicenter Information System (ARAMIS). Their results include the following:

- Gastrointestinal (GI) tract complications associated with NSAIDs are the most common serious adverse drug reactions in the United States.
- NSAID-associated gastropathy (ulcers and bleeding) can be estimated to account for at least 2,600 deaths and 20,000 hospitalizations each year in patients with rheumatoid arthritis alone.
- The rate of complications in patients with rheumatoid arthritis studied prospectively demonstrated that approximately 6 percent per year got into trouble with their NSAIDs, experiencing a significant gastrointestinal side effect with about 1.3 percent of patients requiring hospitalization.
- A large majority of these patients did *not* have GI problems prior to NSAID use, and prophylactic treatment with antacids and H2 blockers were not found to be of value.
- The relative risk of a GI-provoked hospitalization was more than five times greater in patients taking NSAIDs.
- A toxicity index showed buffered aspirin, salsalate and

ibuprofen emerging as the least toxic medications, with tolmetin sodium, meclofenamate and indomethacin as the most toxic.
· The most important risk factors are advanced age, use of the steroid prednisone, previous NSAID GI toxicity, prior GI hospitalization and high functional joint disability (based on American Rheumatology Association classification).

## Nonnarcotic Drugs (Nonopioids)

In severe cases of arthritis doctors may use more powerful pain relievers.

These include steroids which may be taken orally or injected directly into the joints. Ketorolac (Toradol), although an NSAID, is available as an injection and usually gives rapid though short-acting pain relief. Oral tramadol (Ultram) is available for moderate to severe pain. When introduced into the United States market in 1996 from Europe, it was classified by the FDA as a nonnarcotic and considered to have little to no potential for dependence or addiction, yet caution is now being advised in that some cases of addiction have been reported. Also of note is that tramadol has been associated with seizures in susceptible individuals, especially when given at high doses. This risk increases if it is given concurrently with antidepressant drugs such as desipramine (Norpramin) and doxepin (Sinequan). Caution has also been advised with agents known as selective serotonin reuptake inhibitors, including fluoxetine (Prozac), sertraline (Zoloft) and paroxetine (Paxil).

## Narcotic (Opioid) Drugs

Narcotic drugs may also be used for relieving extreme pain (see Table 4.3).

The preferred medical term is *opiate* or *opioid*, rather than *narcotic*, possibly to avoid the suggestion that these medical drugs make one sleepy (the Greek word for sleep is *narcosis*). *Opiates* are specifically those drugs such as morphine and codeine that are physically derived from opium. Most drugs in this family act on the opioid receptors but are semisynthetic or synthetic; hence, these partially or totally synthesized substances are more properly called *opioids*, indicating that they are synthesized as opposed to being naturally derived.

For arthritis, the most commonly used drugs are propoxyphine (Darvon), codeine (Tylenol #3 and #4) and hydrocodone (Vicodin and Lorcet), although oxycodone (Percodan and Percocet), particularly the sustained released form (OxyContin), is increasingly used. These agents may be combined with acetaminophen or aspirin and frequently are sold in fixed combinations. It is important to note that the amount of acetaminophen in a fixed combination may pose significant complications because it is recommended that the daily intake of acetaminophen not exceed four grams. Exceeding this upper limit may cause liver or kidney problems, or both, a warning not to be taken lightly.

While narcotic drugs may facilitate quick pain relief and allow for more activity during the day as well as rest or sleep in cases where pain disrupts rest, these drugs are powerful and are known to cause dependence and, in some cases, addiction. While addiction is uncommon, physicians are rightfully wary of using these drugs on a long-term basis. Prescribing them should be done only when conservative therapies have failed and the patient clearly understands the risks and benefits of long-term use. Careful supervision, preferably by a pain management physician, is warranted, and prescriptions should not be refilled unless the patient is seen face-to-face by the prescribing physician.

Narcotic drugs, however, are being used more and more in advanced osteoarthritis, even more so in the severe inflammatory arthritis disorders (rheumatoid, ankylosing spondylitis, psoriatic arthritis). Most of the time, the weaker or less potent opioids are used and are formulated with either aspirin or acetaminophen. Part of this increasing usage is due to the advocacy position taken by algologists (physicians specializing in pain management), and more recently articulated by a consensus statement from the American Academy of Pain Medicine.[12] Data is abundant that functionality improves and addiction does not occur if a legitimate medical condition—cancer or non-cancer accompanied by severe pain—is treated aggressively within a pain management treatment plan. The intent with opioids as with other pain medication is to enhance sensible activity and improve rest— restoring the patient to a reasonable level of well-being. Even the stronger opiods such as morphine, methadone and sustained-release oxycodone (Oxycontin) are now being used for noncancer pain, including arthritis. Oxycontin, in fact, was recently listed in the *Physicians' Desk Reference* as a possible drug choice for noncancer pain, including arthritis. This was a first for an opioid.

While narcotic drugs may facilitate pain relief, they are not without side effects and significant expense. As physicians, our goal is to prevent pain and disability by early recognition and treatment, primarily with sensible diet and lifestyle changes, using opioids only in advanced disease and under careful supervision.

Physical dependence is a given with opioids, whether they are strong or weak; thus, withdrawal symptoms such as agitation, cold sweats, diarrhea and confusion will occur if they are stopped abruptly. For this reason, the use of these drugs is not to be taken lightly, and only physicians skilled in their management should be regularly dispensing them.

### TABLE 4.3

### NARCOTICS MOST COMMONLY USED FOR ARTHRITIS

| Generic Name | Trade Name |
| --- | --- |
| Codeine with acetaminophen | Tylenol #3, Phenaphen #3 |
| Dihydrocodeine | Synalgos DC, DHC Plus |
| Hydrocodone with acetaminophen | Vicodin, Lorcet, Lortab |
| Methadone | Dolophine |
| Morphine sustained release | Ms Contin, Oramorph, Kadian |
| Oxycodone sustained release | Oxycontin |
| Pentazocine | Talwin |
| Pentazocine with acetaminophen | Talacen |
| Propoxyphene | Darvon |
| Proproxyphene with acetaminophen | Darvocet |
| Propoxyphene with aspirin | Darvon Compound |

There is another class of drugs, known as mixed agonists/antagonists, which should be mentioned. They are synthetic narcotics and they are occasionally used for pain control. These drugs include:

| Generic name | Trade name |
| --- | --- |
| Pentazocine | Talwin-NX, Talacen |
| Nalbuphine | Nubain |
| Butorphanol | Stadol, Stadol NS |
| Buprenorphine | Buprenex |

Only pentazocine is available in oral form and likely to be useful only in some cases of advanced arthritis. The property that these compounds have in common is that they have mixed activity on the narcotic receptors. They will enhance pain relief but only to a certain point. They are said to have a "low ceiling effect," which means that a small amount may be helpful, but if the dose is increased there are likely to be significant complications related to an antagonistic effect on the narcotic receptors. Worse yet, if the patient is given one of these mixed agents when already on a strong narcotic, it can precipitate a withdrawal syndrome. Nalbuphine, butorphanol and buprenorphine are available only in injectable form. For the pain associated with labor and delivery, nalbuphine (Nubain) and butorphanol (Stadol) are used frequently, but they are best avoided for treating arthritis. Note that butorphanol also is available in a nasal spray (Stadol NS) that is being marketed primarily for migraine headaches. For arthritis, however, it is best to avoid this drug.

## Cortisone Medications

The most powerful anti-inflammatory drugs are the cortisone-type medications or corticosteroids. They can be life-saving when given for acute asthma or adrenal crisis. They may provide complete pain relief when given in high doses on a short-term basis for patients with rheumatoid arthritis flare-ups or when injected into a painful, red-hot, swollen joint. Doctors try to eliminate their serious side effects by giving as low a dose as possible and using injections at the site of inflammation.

However, these drugs should be used only as the very last resort because of their significant long-term side effects which include osteoporosis and fractures; cataracts; glaucoma; high blood pressure; stomach irritation and bleeding; weight gain; frequent infections; and worsening of diabetes mellitus.

## Antibiotics

Occasionally, we find antibiotics recommended for some forms of inflammatory arthritis because of potential bacterial etiologies. The use of antibiotics can increase risk for serious yeast infection and cause an imbalance of the body's flora required for the proper digestion and synthesis of nutrients from foods. However, their use may be indicated if natural healing pathways for supporting immune function don't seem to work alone. If antibiotics are used, be sure to use a quality probiotic acidophilus supplement or organic yogurt with various friendly bacterial cultures and fructooligosaccharides (which stimulate the growth of friendly bacteria) to help in recultivating the body's bacterial balance.

## Problems with NSAIDs

As previously stated, instances do occur when the use of these drugs is the best course of action. However, in the case of arthritis, we believe that the use of these drugs without first trying glucosamine sulfate to be medical treatment in the most narrow sense.

As early as 1978 researchers from Rotta Research Laboratories (Milano, Italy) reported NSAIDs actually inhibit the body's ability to produce its cartilage matrix. They pointed out that the metabolism of the cartilage may even be impaired and the degenerative process accelerated using these drugs. Nonsteroidal anti-inflammatory agents, they asserted, should be given only for a short period time when pain is very severe.

Meanwhile researchers, writing in *Current Medical Research and Opinion*, note:

> Most of [the typically prescribed drugs] have proved to reduce the metabolic capacity of the cartilage, and this could lead possibly to an impairment of articular function in the long run. Most of these preparations, moreover, cannot be administered as long as necessary, either because of inconvenience to the patient or because of severe side effects, usually gastric.[13]

In that same journal, José M. Pujalte, M.D., and coinvestigators concluded that, "In the long run this could result in an even worse condition."[14]

This finding of a poorer state of joint health after the use of common arthritis drugs has been verified in many studies published in journals such as *Lancet* and the *Journal of Bone and Joint Surgery*.[15-17] Preliminary clinical data suggest a method of action by which ibuprofen-type drugs may have a negative effect on joint health: they adversely affect the body's balance of prostaglandins, the family of fatty acids involved in the body's inflammation and healing processes.[18]

Although NSAIDS reduce the signs and symptoms of osteoarthritis and rheumatoid arthritis and bring relief to millions of people, they "do not eliminate underlying disease. Disease-modifying antirheumatic drugs also bring relief, but these drugs are often ineffective and not well tolerated. Failure to provide long-term benefits combined with the high toxicity of most of the disease-modifying agents has prompted a search for more effective treatments," wrote Dr. G. Spencer-Green in a 1993 issue of *Postgraduate Medicine*.[19]

Drugs used in the treatment of osteoarthritis and rheumatoid arthritis (including probably dexamethasone) also have the potential of depleting the blood of another important nutrient, sulfate, which, as we shall see more thoroughly in Chapter 6, is necessary to the body's production of cartilage cells called glycosaminoglycans.

Indeed, the body is already not producing enough sulfur-derived glycosaminoglycans, the building blocks of cartilage, when it is suffering from osteoarthritis. Under the influence of NSAIDs, the body produces even fewer glycosaminoglycans. Those that are produced tend to be sulfate-depleted and inferior in quality. This results in further joint deterioration and is intrinsically in opposition to healing.

Yet, because humans naturally have very low serum sulfate levels in their blood, they react extremely sensitively to sulfate depletion. Thus, the very drugs intended to help damage the joint even more by depleting the body of sulfate.

Glucosamine sulfate, on the other hand, while it doesn't work as fast as these pain killers, preserves the body's delicate sulfate balance, and actually seems to work better after the first week or two of use, providing a deeper, longer lasting period of pain relief and, of course, stimulating joint regeneration.

### DON'T MASK PAIN

*If you do use pain killers, be sure not to use them before exercising just to get a better workout. If you mask pain, you'll never know when you are doing damage. Use pain killers, if at all, only **after** exercise.*

Unlike NSAIDs, cortisone-type medications and other drugs— other medical treatments for osteoarthritis *are* safe and helpful. The trouble is, they may not be able to make up for the long-term joint deterioration that often accompanies various forms of arthritis. These safe and somewhat effective pain treatments include the use of moist heat or cold packs, exercise, stretching and weight loss when necessary. We believe that these are excellent strategies, although most rheumatologists and their patients tend not to place enough emphasis on diet, exercise, weight loss and nutritional supplements, instead preferring to prescribe the types of drugs that we have discussed in this chapter.

## Bottom Line

- NSAIDs offer quick pain relief, but they do not address the underlying condition, and may even hasten the degeneration of the joint.
- If you must use NSAIDs for quick pain relief, try to avoid their use beyond two or three days.
- After that, try glucosamine sulfate in three divided doses daily of 500 mg each.
- If you are a long-term user of NSAIDs or other drugs, work with your doctor or health professional to gradually taper your dosage of these drugs.

# PART II

# 5
# Joint Anatomy

The body's joints are truly amazing. The biomechanical union of two bones in the body, a smoothly moving healthy joint's mobility far exceeds that of mechanical engineering's even greatest feats. The joints glide and rotate using the most lubricating, water-based ecology ever invented.

Human joints rotate, go forward, backward, even side to side. Think about your knee's freedom of movement or that of your fingers, especially your thumb. Every movement you make is the result of your joints' mobility. Running, jumping, hopping, sewing, knitting, dancing, hiking, even painting are all possible thanks to your body's joints. Your joints help to make you, physically, fully dimensional.

Such natural smoothness depends on properly nourished joint surfaces. An amazing fact about joints: they have no blood vessels. The joints are encapsulated within a watery envelope and consist of a synovium membrane, synovial fluids, ligaments, tendons and muscles bathed in nutrient-rich liquid within the capsule. These living permeable tissues rely on the body's movements, its inner tides, for their nourishment and health. Their delicate watery balance gives way to bone scraping if nourishment doesn't reach the joint tissues, and cartilage becomes worn and unrepaired without proper nourishment and maintenance.

*Every movement you make is the result of your joints'*
*mobility. Running, jumping, hopping, sewing, knitting,*
*dancing, hiking, even painting are all possible thanks*
*to your body's joints. Your joints help to make you,*
*physically, fully dimensional.*

### Types of Joints

*There are three major types of joints:*
· The sutures in your skull: relatively fixed joints.
· The sacroiliac and spinal vertebrae: slightly movable joints.
· The wrists, knees, and neck: highly movable joints.

## Cartilage—A Closer Look

Imagine tennis shoes without cushioning. Imagine playing basketball on concrete. Imagine jogging on a hard concrete pavement. If your cartilage remains healthy, these images will remain figments of your imagination. If your cartilage becomes diseased and requires healing, as in arthritis, your joints and legs will cry out in pain.

Cartilage is the firm, white connective tissue at the end of bones. Have you ever looked at the ends of a chicken bone? The blue-white, shiny stuff is cartilage. Cartilage is known as the body's shock absorber and it works extremely well even though we probably start to lose some of our body's abundant reserves in our teens. Cartilage is more slippery than ice; its ecology is up to

80 percent water. Because it does not have blood vessels it must be nourished through fluid exchange.

Articular cartilage, at the ends of bones, is a specialized form of connective tissue. This is the type of cartilage usually involved in osteoarthritis and rheumatoid arthritis. It is extremely slippery—some eight times more slippery than ice.

Articular cartilage is made up of collagen, proteoglycans, chondrocytes and water. Let's look at each of these components a little more closely.

**Collagen** is made up of densely woven strands of amino acids built into chains of proteins. Collagen might be aptly called the threads of cartilage. It imparts shape and resiliency to cartilage. The type of collagen in cartilage is a very unique and special collagen found only in cartilage. It is called collagen type II.

**Proteoglycans** are large, water-loving molecules made from protein and sugar. They are interwoven into the collagen. When healthy, proteoglycans look like fresh Christmas trees; when they are diseased, as with osteoarthritis, they resemble the dried-out, cast-off Christmas leftovers consigned to the side of the road for the trash collector.

A water-loving mortar-like material, proteoglycans hold the threads of collagen together and help to nurture cartilage—like tiny irrigation canals. Proteoglycans, strung together, impart shape, size and resiliency to cartilage. The water-loving proteoglycans and collagen are responsible for the biomechanical and biochemical properties making articular cartilage unique in its function as gliding surface *and* shock absorber for the joints.

Sprinkled within this matrix outside of the cells are tiny, cartilage factories called the **chondrocytes**. These powerhouse cells are the only living element in cartilage and are like the brains *and* workers of the joints. They produce proteoglycans and collagen molecules so that cartilage remains healthy and cushioning. When proteoglycans and collagen are worn out, the chondrocytes release enzymes that eat up and digest those that are most weakened.

The body's supply of proteoglycans and collagen is governed by the health of its chondrocytes. If, due to toxicity, malnutrition, immune responses or other biological processes, the chondrocytes start dying faster than they can be regenerated, the mortar-like material that makes up cartilage is left unrepaired because there is nothing there to order the job done. Then, cartilage falls into a state of disrepair.

When cartilage is healthy, the articular cartilage is white, smooth and firm to the touch. Microscopically, it shows strong color variations (metachromasia) due to the high proteoglycan content. Beneath the abundant proteoglycans, cartilage appears threaded due to the interwoven collagen, which relieves the compression and traction forces caused by body movements.

In the first stages of osteoarthritis, the cartilage appears faded and the beautiful metachromasia of health is yielding. Inside the body, the cartilage releases proteoglycans into the synovial fluid and gradually loses its metachromatic appearance. It hardly resists the compressive forces, and the fibrous network previously masked by proteoglycans is progressively revealed. The biomechanical effect also involves the fibrous collagen framework. Collagen fibers splinter, releasing their elemental building fibrils in a process known as fibrillation. The chondrocytes also become damaged, leading to progressive cell distress and eventually tissue death.

Over time, the cartilage slowly cracks, turning rough and pitted, like the sun-baked, cracked, drought-blighted desert earth. Flecks and bits of cartilage break off and can end up in the joint fluid, irritating the synovium membrane and causing pain.

If left untreated, arthritis worsens into joint degeneration. The cartilage wears down and synovial fluids leak into areas of the cartilage. The fluid leaks toxic, cartilage-destroying enzymes (collagenases and proteoglyconases) into the cartilage. Gradually, these cartilage-damaging enzymes outpower joint protectors. These molecular sharks cause further joint deterioration.

If the body's healing mechanism is overwhelmed, cartilage will eventually wear through and leave the bone exposed. The body tries to compensate, and emergency blood vessels grow into an area that once had none. The area is now a stressed ecosystem within the body. Repair processes are poor, and the new cartilage is supported with inferior mortar that enjoys only a short lifetime. The new surface, called fibrocartilage, is also inferior. It is the last layer masking the bone, and small bits of bone already may be poking through. Mineralized osteophytes grow like rude stalactites on the ends of the afflicted bone. These cause scraping or break off and irritate synovial membranes even further.

"Gradually this cartilage becomes thinner and roughened," observes medical editor Charles Clayman, M.D., in *The Human Body*. "When the bone underneath the cartilage eventually erodes, bone surfaces rub directly against one another, causing severe discomfort."

Now, the bones become extremely inflamed, as synovial fluid and toxins leak into the marrow in ever greater amounts, causing further destruction.

The situation eventually can be crippling, making movement difficult, if not impossible. Until glucosamine sulfate came onto the scene, nothing, in fact, could be done to regenerate cartilage. Indeed, one very important role of glucosamine sulfate is the inhibition of cartilage-degrading enzymes. In a recent test tube study performed with human osteoarthritis cartilage, it was demonstrated that glucosamine sulfate is able to inhibit collagenase, the key enzyme in osteoarthritis cartilage destruction, and also cellular phospholipase A2, an activator of collagenase, resulting in a complete suppression of collagenase activity.[20]

In other words, glucosamine sulfate may be the best news tired, aching joints have ever had.

Now let's look at the studies that support glucosamine sulfate's use in arthritis and what these studies say about its effectiveness for the average consumer who seeks safe regeneration of the joints and freedom from pain.

# 6
# Reversal of Arthritis and Degenerative Joints with Glucosamine Sulfate

When looking for a medical therapy, it is best whenever possible, to find one that changes the underlying state of disease; one that actually emphasizes healing rather than just relieving symptoms.

Up to now, in the case of arthritis, even though patients' symptoms could be alleviated with aspirin or other NSAIDs, the pain always came back, and the underlying cause was never addressed. Indeed, research has shown that long-term use of NSAIDs may actually impair healing and damage joint cartilage further.

According to Professor L. Rovati, president of Rotta Research Laboratories which has performed the bulk of the world's glucosamine sulfate research, the study of glucosamine dates to the late 19th century when it was first discovered.

Glucosamine is a member of the glycosaminoglycan family.[21] Glycosaminoglycans are long chains of amino acids (or proteins) that are found in high concentration in sea shells, from which glucosamine is harvested. Glucosamine sulfate is a natural aminosugar. A simple, very small molecule composed of glucose, glutamine and sulfur, it is highly soluble in water. Glucosamine sulfate is now known to be used by the body to manufacture proteoglycans, which, as you may recall, hold the collagen threads together and retain the water necessary to import shape, size and resiliency to collagen. Early on, researchers discovered that healthy joint cartilage has high concentrations of glucosamine sulfate.

The early work on glucosamine sulfate attempted to ascertain both its safety and principles of action. Most of these studies were of a preliminary nature and are what we refer to as *in vitro* or test tube studies.

By the 1950s, researchers were employing a variety of culture media, incubation times and types of fibroblasts (cells that contribute to the formation of connective tissue fibers) or cartilage samples from different sources, using different determination methods to evaluate the effects of glucosamine sulfate on actual biological tissues.[22]

Researchers began by actually growing cartilage tissue in a test tube. Then they put NSAIDs with cartilage cells in one dish and glucosamine sulfate with identical cartilage cells in another dish. What they found was amazing. The NSAIDs damaged the cartilage cells while the glucosamine sulfate actually stimulated more healthy cartilage regrowth. This was very important because it was concrete evidence that showed glucosamine sulfate could actually modify disease. Subsequent studies showed that glucosamine could penetrate intact articular cartilage within the human body. After intravenous and oral administration, glucosamine sulfate was found to be enriched in cartilage tissues.[23, 24]

Researchers also examined the primary components of glucosamine sulfate: glucose, glutamine and sulfate, as these each have important roles in the metabolism of the body's joints.

In 1951, researchers, using radioactive tagging, discovered that the sulfate portion was actually taken up by the joints and converted into glycosaminoglycans.[25] Again, this is extremely important because glycosaminoglycans are building blocks for the body's supply of proteoglycans.

In 1974, research demonstrated that increasing concentrations of radioactively tagged glucosamine stimulated increased glycosaminoglycan production when added to cultured chick embryo cartilage.[26]

These findings were confirmed in 1978 when glucosamine was conclusively shown to stimulate glycosaminoglycan production in cultured mouse tissues.[22]

These results were amplified by a human tissue study published in 1979 in the *Journal of Bone and Joint Surgery*. Changes in rates of glycosaminoglycan synthesis were studied in 37 samples of actual human articular cartilage from both people with osteoarthritis and from normal control patients 50 to 75 years old.[27] The samples from people with the worst cases of osteoarthritis showed significantly depleted levels of glycosaminoglycans in their cartilage. In fact, the greater the loss, the worse the condition. The researchers theorized that glucosamine, which stimulates the body's production of glycosaminoglycans, could help to rejuvenate cartilage.

By enhancing the body's supply of these important proteoglycan building blocks, glucosamine sulfate induces a dose-dependent stimulation of the production of complete proteoglycans identical to those found in human cartilage. By the 1980s, glucosamine sulfate appeared to also be a valid means to fight the chondrocyte deficiency that typically develops during osteoarthritis.

Glucosamine sulfate actually feeds the joints and stimulates regrowth (at the cellular level) of the materials that comprise cartilage. The healing miracle of glucosamine sulfate, then, we now know, is that its ingestion stimulates the body to manufacture more proteoglycans or cartilage matrix, returning a healthy strength and integrity to the joints. Glucosamine sulfate is the first totally safe joint-regenerating substance to be available to the public without a prescription.

Another powerful attribute of glucosamine sulfate is its ability to inhibit cartilage-degrading enzymes.

Luke Bucci, Ph.D., reports in his book *Pain Free* that glucosamine "is the single most important component and precursor for [glycosaminoglycans]," which support the body's population of proteoglycans and other substances that make up the cartilage matrix. "Collagen production also requires glucosamine," Bucci reports. However, "during joint degeneration and arthritis, chondrocytes have been 'told' to destroy cartilage. Manufacture of new cartilage cannot keep pace with the destruction." Glucosamine favorably turns the tide, restimulating production of proteoglycans.[28]

As one team of researchers notes,

> Indeed, altered glucosamine metabolism would appear to be part of the background of arthrosis and, according to recent biochemical and pharmacological findings, the administration of glucosamine tends to normalize cartilage metabolism, so as to inhibit the degradation and stimulate the synthesis of proteoglycans and, finally, to restore, at least partially, the articular function. Animal studies have shown that orally administered glucosamine is taken up selectively by cartilage.[13]

That is why glucosamine is a healing food for damaged joints.

*Glucosamine sulfate actually feeds the joints and stimulates regrowth at the cellular level. It is the first totally safe joint-regenerating substance to be widely available to the public without a prescription.*

GLUCOSAMINE SULFATE WORKS IN THE FOLLOWING WAYS . . .

- *As joint food (the actual building block of cartilage).*
- *Prevents cartilage breakdown.*
- *Rebuilds cartilage.*
- *Provides long-lasting pain relief.*

The scientific studies that validate modern glucosamine sulfate therapies now cover more than four decades, starting with fundamental test tube studies, animal modeling and pharmacokinetic investigations (the study of how substances are absorbed, their metabolic pathways and potential toxicity) in addition to subsequent human clinical trials.[29]

These studies have been performed in Germany, Italy, Spain, Portugal, France and China. Presently, long-term studies are being conducted in Belgium and the Slovak Republic. They are being carried out on people suffering many forms of osteoarthritis. In total, more than 6,000 patients have been studied.[30]

Once the safety of glucosamine sulfate was ascertained, it was time for the research to progress to human clinical trials. These studies also led to the refinement of a patented form of glucosamine sulfate from Rotta Research Laboratories, eventually registered with the United States Patent Office on February 10, 1987.

The human studies, progressing from small and preliminary to major multicenter randomized tests, began around 1980. Some of the clinical trials were classic double-blind, placebo-controlled tests. Others compared glucosamine sulfate to familiar painkilling drugs such as ibuprofen. Many studies are on-going as we write. We have reviewed the entire set of published studies, looking specifically at orally delivered glucosamine sulfate and have selected many to study closely. The following studies are typical of many others cited in the literature.

**#1.** One of the earliest studies was a small-scale pilot study reported in 1980 in *Current Medical Research and Opinion*. Drs. G. Crolle and E. D'Este, of the G.B. Giustinian Hospital, Venice, Italy, gave two groups of 15 patients with osteoarthritis either 400 mg of pure glucosamine sulfate daily by intramuscular injection for seven days followed by two weeks of 1.5 grams daily oral glucosamine sulfate in three divided doses or the painkilling drugs piperazine/chlorbutanol followed by oral placebo during the following two weeks.[30]

The patients' improvement was measured for pain at rest and during active and passive movements, range of function and walking time over 20 meters. They were tested before and after one and three weeks of treatment. The researchers reported that in spite of the short period of treatment, a "substantial proportion of the patients treated with glucosamine sulfate became symptom-free." Three patients (20 percent) in the group receiving glucosamine sulfate felt better after the first week of treatment, and one more (totaling 27 percent) felt great after the maintenance period.

"None of the patients given the comparative treatment was reported as symptom-free, at any time. . . . It was highly significant from the clinical point of view, mainly because our patients with chronic arthrosis were of advanced age and usually with concurrent severe ailments."[29]

The group receiving piperazine/chlorbutanol drugs had an initial reduction in symptoms, but lost all of their gains after the first week. At about the same time, for the patients receiving the oral dose of glucosamine sulfate, the effects of the treatment began to kick in. They began showing rapid improvement in scores such as pain at rest, pain on active movement and other function and walking measurements.

## Symptom Scores Before and During the G.B. Giustinian Hospital Study[30]

| Assessment | Time | Glucosamine Group | Reference Group |
|---|---|---|---|
| Pain at rest | 0 | 1.71 | 1.50 |
| | 7 | 0.36 | 0.63 |
| | 21 | 0.21 | 1.13 |
| Pain on active | 0 | 2.53 | 2.21 |
| movement | 7 | 0.93 | 1.00 |
| | 21 | 0.67 | 1.86 |
| Pain on passive | 0 | 1.80 | 1.14 |
| movement | 7 | 0.27 | 0.50 |
| | 21 | 0.20 | 1.07 |
| Restricted | 0 | 1.69 | 1.86 |
| function | 7 | 0.62 | 1.14 |
| | 21 | 0.38 | 1.71 |
| Time to walk (20 | 0 | 49.6 | 40.4 |
| meters) | 7 | 36.0 | 31.5 |
| | 21 | 28.6 | 38.9 |

**#2.** Pilot studies begat larger studies. Another study that year had almost three times the number of enrolled participants. The study was published in 1980 by A. Drovani of the Vigevano General Hospital and co-researchers in *Clinical Therapeutics*.[31]

In this study, oral administration was used. Since most people only have the oral form of glucosamine sulfate available to them over the counter, this is the fairest representation for the average medical consumer.

Eighty patients with osteoarthritis were given 1.5 grams of glucosamine sulfate, as with previous studies from Rotta Research Laboratories, in three divided oral doses for 30 days. Articular pain, joint tenderness and swelling and restriction of active and passive movements were scored at one-week intervals.

The authors reported that patients treated with glucosamine sulfate experienced a reduction in overall symptoms "almost twice as large (73 percent vs. 41 percent) and twice as fast (time to reduce symptoms by 50 percent: 20 days vs. 36 days) as those who had placebo."[31] Effects, they emphasized, were "impressively superior to placebo."

Samples of articular cartilage were obtained from several patients as part of their normal medical care. These were examined by scanning electron microscopy, a procedure by which researchers look very closely at the surface of the cartilage. The glucosamine group's cartilage was much smoother and less rough or pitted than those receiving placebo. The cartilage of treated women with severe cartilage damage had become almost smooth without the major irregularities of the diseased tissue. *The glucosamine sulfate treatment appeared to have entirely rebuilt the cartilage.*

Joint function increased rapidly and effectively, they observed. In fact, they wrote, a "substantial percentage of patients completely regained their mobility. . . . A longer treatment would result in an even greater proportion of success in patients with

### Patient Improvement Scores During Vigevano General Study[31]

| Relief of Symptoms | Number of Patients Receiving | |
| --- | --- | --- |
| | Glucosamine Sulfate | Placebo |
| Pain and tenderness | 10/40 | 0/40 |
| Restriction of active and passive movements | 9/40 | 0/40 |
| Overall symptoms | 8/40 | 0/40 |

chronic illness . . ." In fact eight of the 40 patients receiving the glucosamine sulfate became symptom-free while none of the placebo group did.

**#3.** Now the published data from the clinical trials began coming in quickly. The two studies in 1980 were followed by several more. In each case, the studies strongly supported the use of oral glucosamine sulfate for healing osteoarthritis, especially in the most intractable, unresponsive cases.

In 1981, E. d'Ambrosio and coinvestigators carried out their glucosamine sulfate work at G. Stuard Hospital, Parma, Italy. They detailed their study of 30 patients with chronic, degenerative osteoarthritis in *Pharmatherapeutica*. The glucosamine sulfate therapy outperformed the typical drug therapy and with complete safety.

> In conclusion, the results of this short-term study in a limited number of patients indicate that this new preparation containing pure glucosamine sulphate is an effective and very well-tolerated treatment for arthrosis. . . . In our experience, treatment with glucosamine sulphate resulted in a further increase in the improvement already obtained . . .
> *Since glucosamine sulphate is also extremely well tolerated, has no contra-indications and no interactions with other drugs, it would appear to be a drug of first choice for the basic and long-term treatment of primary or secondary osteoarthrosic disorders.*[32]

**#4.** Osteoarthritis of the knee is always troubling and can often require surgery or extremely potent OTC drugs such as ibuprofen. Could glucosamine sulfate improve symptoms and therefore reduce dependence on more toxic pharmaceutical drugs?

In 1982, a double-blind trial was done on 40 outpatients with osteoarthritis of the knee to compare the efficacy, safety and

## Symptom Scores Before and During the G. Stuard Hospital Study[32]

| Symptom | Day | Glucosamine Group | Reference Group |
|---|---|---|---|
| Pain at rest | 0 | 1.80 | 1.86 |
|  | 7 | 0.53 | 1.13 |
|  | 21 | 0.33 | 1.20 |
| Pain during active | 0 | 2.22 | 1.93 |
| movement | 7 | 0.93 | 1.26 |
|  | 21 | 0.73 | 1.40 |
| Pain during | 0 | 2.13 | 1.93 |
| passive | 7 | 0.93 | 1.33 |
| movement | 21 | 0.66 | 1.33 |
| Function limitation | 0 | 2.06 | 1.86 |
|  | 7 | 1.06 | 1.53 |
|  | 21 | 0.66 | 1.66 |

tolerance for oral treatment of either the standard amount of glucosamine sulfate (1.5 grams) or 1.2 grams of ibuprofen for eight weeks.[33]

This study comparing glucosamine to ibuprofen was analogous to having two of America's best professional football teams compete on Super Bowl Sunday. Ibuprofen is no slouch when it comes to pain relief; could glucosamine sulfate actually knock off this proven pain reliever? At first it looked as though ibuprofen was going to cash in on a stunning victory. Antonio Lopes Vaz, M.D., of St. John Hospital, Oporto, Portugal, found that at first the patients' "pain scores decreased faster during the first two weeks in the ibuprofen than in the glucosamine treatment group."

Over the long run, however, the glucosamine sulfate group proved the winner. "Although the rate of decrease was slower, the reduction in pain scores was continued throughout the trial period in patients on glucosamine, and the difference between the two groups turned significantly in favor of glucosamine at week 8."

**#5.** Another study in 1982 proved to be the largest to date and greatly advanced the European community's faith in glucosamine sulfate as a safe healing and pain-relieving front line treatment for osteoarthritis. M.J. Tapadinhas and coinvestigators published their study in 1982 in *Pharmatherapeutica*.[34] This ambitious project was undertaken at treatment centers among some 1,500 osteoarthritis patients throughout Portugal. Their ages were 16 to 84, with an average age of 52.

More than half had other conditions aggravating their osteoarthritis. This trial with so many people also tested whether glucosamine sulfate interacted with other medications taken for such conditions as depression, obesity, diabetes, heart and kidney disease. No drug interactions were reported.

Moreover, some 110 people who had shown no improvement from any other treatment responded dramatically to glucosamine sulfate. In total, some 95 percent of the patients had good results, substantially higher than the 70-percent rate for drugs such as ibuprofen, also being studied.

Glucosamine sulfate "manages most arthrosis patients to full or partial recovery, whatever the localization of their arthrosis, concomitant illnesses or treatments . . ."[34]

**#6.** Moving into the 1990s, L.C. Rovati, from the Department of Clinical Pharmacology, Rotta Research Laboratories, reported in *International Journal of Tissue Reactions* that three double-blind, controlled, parallel group studies were being carried out.[35] A total of 606 people with osteoarthritis were scored for improvements in mobility, including active and passive movement, according to all of the standard measurement protocols established and used in earlier studies.

"Glucosamine was significantly more effective than placebo, while no difference was detected in comparison with NSAIDs," the report noted. "On the other hand, glucosamine was as well-tolerated as placebo, while the percentage of patients suffering adverse drug reactions was higher in the ibuprofen group."

Indeed, more than one-third of the NSAID users had bad reactions to the drugs.

**#7.** In 1994, in *Osteoarthritis and Cartilage*, Wolfgang Noack of the Department of Orthopedics at Berlin's *Waldrankenhaus* and coinvestigators reported results of their multicenter placebo-controlled, double-blind study involving 252 outpatients with osteoarthritis of the knee.[36] Patients were treated with either placebo or oral glucosamine sulfate at 1.5 grams for four weeks with weekly clinic visits. The patients receiving glucosamine sulfate had substantially lower pain scores than those who received only the placebo.

"We have shown that oral glucosamine sulfate (1500 mg/day) was significantly more effective than placebo in improving pain and movement limitation in patients with OA of the knee."[36]

## Pain Relief Measurements at Weekly Intervals[36]

| Week | Pain Relief Score Glucosamine Sulfate | Pain Relief Score Placebo |
|---|---|---|
| 0 | 10.6 | 10.6 |
| 1 | 10.0 | 10.1 |
| 2 | 8.8 | 9.3 |
| 3 | 7.9 | 8.6 |
| 4 | 7.4 | 8.4 |

**#8.** Also in 1994, Rovati reported on a large, randomized, placebo-controlled, double-blind study comparing glucosamine sulfate to the very popular NSAID, piroxicam (Feldene). Although helpful in reducing pain, some 40 percent of users suffered complications.[37] In France, 41 percent of the people taking piroxicam experienced side effects, especially stomach bleeding and ulcers, the researchers reported.

The 329 patients were given either the standard 1.5 gram dosage of glucosamine sulfate or 20 mg of piroxicam, both or placebo.

In the study, glucosamine sulfate outperformed piroxicam. The researchers concluded:

> Glucosamine sulfate was confirmed as an effective, well-tolerated, symptomatic, slow-acting drug in osteoarthritis, with a steadily increasing effect, persisting after drug withdrawal. Piroxicam was less tolerated, had a similar efficacy at the beginning of treatment, wore off at withdrawal.[37]

Though glucosamine sulfate was also paired with piroxicam, the glucosamine sulfate given alone produced even better results.

**#9.** Another rematch between ibuprofen and glucosamine was arranged, the results of which were published in 1994 in *Osteoarthritis and Cartilage*.

The study team, led by German-based researcher Hans Müller-Faβender and coscientists included 200 hospitalized patients with osteoarthritis of the knee for three months or longer. The patients were divided into two groups of about 100 each.[38]

The improvement occurred sooner in the ibuprofen group, but no difference in pain relief between the two was reported from the second week onward, reported the authors. Both groups ended up statistically even in terms of pain relief, but the glucosamine group actually enjoyed longer-lasting, deeper healing.

"Glucosamine sulfate was therefore as effective as ibuprofen for alleviating symptoms of knee OA," they wrote.

Thirty-five out of 100 patients using ibuprofen complained of side effects, particularly of the gastrointestine. Seven dropped out. Only six of 100 in the glucosamine group complained; one dropped out.

### Adverse Events Reported During Study (Glucosamine Sulfate vs. Ibuprofen)[38]

| Adverse Event | Glucosamine Sulfate | Ibuprofen |
|---|---|---|
| Gastrointestinal complaints | 5 (1) | 29 (4) |
| Pruritus or skin reactions | 1 (0) | 4 (3) |
| Flushing | 0 (0) | 1 (0) |
| Fatigue | 0 (0) | 1 (0) |
| Total | 6 (1) | 35 (7) |

The figure in parentheses is the number of drop-outs related to adverse events.

**#10.** In March 1996, N. Giordano and coscientists reported in *Clinica Terapeutica* that their year-long study of glucosamine sulfate's effects on patients with arthritis showed it had a significant protective effect on the chondrocytes.[39]

## In Summary

The earliest studies on glucosamine sulfate date to test tube studies in the 1950s. The research required to develop glucosamine sulfate into a clinically useful health ally has been conducted steadily since. The studies that we reviewed constitute about a third of the number studied in the clinical trials. In total, clinical trials have looked at more than 6,000 patients with osteoarthritis at all major points (knee, hip, hand, spine), mostly over short-term periods, but in some instances over several months or years of treatment. Virtually all of this research was done or supported by Rotta Research Laboratories, which used their patented, stabilized form of glucosamine sulfate.

Multiple lines of evidence from test tube studies, animal modeling and clinical trials have produced extremely heartening, positive results. Glucosamine sulfate has been proven to be a major joint-rebuilding nutrient with minimal risks.

*Joanne, a 52-year-old medical transcriptionist, found that her hands were gradually getting stiff. She began taking aspirin every morning upon awakening. At first, she took only a couple. Eventually, she switched to four enterically coated tablets after realizing that the plain aspirin upset her stomach and made it difficult to eat breakfast. She took another four at her first morning break and then found herself adding acetaminophen to this mixture later in the day.* Yet it still wasn't enough.

*Her line counts were down, and her error rate increased dramatically.*

*Fortunately, one of the physicians for whom she was doing transcriptions was giving his patients glucosamine sulfate. As she was doing their transcriptions, she observed that these patients seemed to be getting better.*

*Joanne made an appointment with the doctor. She was put on glucosamine sulfate, taking 500 mg three times a day. Within two weeks, she noted definite improvement. She felt less early morning stiffness, and the number of aspirins she was taking went down.*

*On her next doctor's visit, she asked her doctor whether she should increase her dosage. The doctor explained to her that more was not necessarily better. Rather, her doctor explained, she should 1) gradually increase her exercise; 2) avoid foods such as beef and dairy, that are high in saturated fats; 3) replace corn and other polyunsaturated oils with olive or flaxseed oil; and 4) pay attention to her stress levels.*

*Two months later, she was completely off aspirin and acetaminophen. Her morning stiffness disappeared, her line counts improved, and her error rate dropped.*

## What About Rheumatoid Arthritis?

In many ways, rheumatoid arthritis is an almost entirely different disease than osteoarthritis. In Chapters 7 and 9, we will discuss the foods and supplemental nutrients that could be key players in relieving the pain of rheumatoid arthritis and that, in some cases, may even initiate the healing process within the body's inflammatory and immune systems.

Glucosamine sulfate was tested in rats in an experimental model of subacute inflammation in both mechanical and immunologically reactive arthritis (which approximates rheumatoid).[40] In both types, glucosamine sulfate "was found effective in oral daily doses." Based on this research, the author opined that glucosamine sulfate "can therefore be considered as a drug of choice for prolonged oral treatment of rheumatic disorders." We believe that glucosamine sulfate is important for people with rheumatoid arthritis to use, because it will help to protect their joints from some of the degenerative effects of this inflammatory condition. Other nutrients also appear to be extremely important, particularly fish oils and combination oral enzymes, as we discuss later.

# If Glucosamine Is So Good,
# Why Doesn't My Doctor Know About It?

In a May 1994 report in the leading scientific journal *Medical Hypotheses*, M.F. McCarty noted that even though many double-blind studies have now been conducted that demonstrate glucosamine sulfate is perhaps the safest, most effective joint-healing nutrient now available, "Medical researchers and physicians in the U.S. have totally ignored this rational and safe therapeutic strategy."[41]

Doctors are often restricted by insurance billing forms and procedures and may also have a prejudice against studies from countries outside of the United States. Also, doctors learn next to nothing about nutrition in medical school. The use of herbs and other natural healing agents is foreign to their practice. "When patients visit their physicians, they expect the visit to end in a transaction which usually involves giving them a prescription to be filled," admits one doctor in speaking of the pressures put on doctors by their patients to prescribe—prescribe anything, just so long as the patient can leave with something tangible, though not always beneficial in the long run.

They may be just plain too busy treating patients to go through research papers and other journals with any kind of depth. They may not subscribe to the newsletters that would quickly bring them up-to-date about recent research. Many doctors simply don't read journals or attend medical meetings. Their primary source of education is pharmaceutical company drug-detail salespersons. Whatever seminars or other educational events they do attend are most likely to be sponsored by pharmaceutical companies which are in the business of selling drugs. Moreover, the great body of glucosamine research is not published in American but European journals, and most U.S. doctors don't read these.

Then there are the insurance companies. By limiting the prescription of natural remedies, some are stifling health freedoms by keeping doctors from practicing safe and healthy medicine. Amazingly, in California, doctors who work for some HMOs are *not* allowed to inform patients of alternative treatments.

However, we believe that HMOs and other insurers will find glucosamine sulfate actually improves their bottom line by keeping their customers healthy and out of the doctor's office. HMOs make money by *not* seeing their patients. HMOs do not pay for nutritional supplements. Yet, ironically, they usually have newsletters advocating supplements. If they can reduce visits or delay them, they make money. Therefore, HMOs are potentially a friend and capable of being friendly toward the use of glucosamine sulfate.

Bucci reports in *Pain Free*,

At this time, the FDA does not accept foreign studies for approval of a new drug in the United States. Also, since glucosamine is already a nutrient, it is very difficult from a legal perspective to file an application to make glucosamine into a drug. . . . You probably won't see glucosamine as an approved drug in this country for many years. This does not mean that glucosamine does not work or is illegal.[28]

However, even if doctors continue to ignore glucosamine sulfate, other more objective organizations have certainly taken note. In 1993, in order to better classify those drugs regarded as selective for osteoarthritis and previously improperly included among the so-called "chondroprotectors" along with other pharmacologically dubious substances, the International League

Against Rheumatism and the World Health Organization coined the acronym SADOA (slow-acting drugs for osteoarthritis), for drugs that "act progressively" compared to symptomatic drugs such as NSAIDs. Glucosamine sulfate is the first such selective drug with a profile that complies with this classification, and only Rotta Research Laboratories' glucosamine sulfate was recently recognized by the International League Against Rheumatism, which has classified it as an accepted "Slow-acting Drug in Osteoarthritis."[2]

## Dosage

The standard dose of glucosamine sulfate is 1.5 grams divided into two to three doses daily, taken after a meal in 500 mg capsules. A powdered form of glucosamine sulfate, which can be mixed into juice, is expected to soon be available. See Resources.

# Choosing a Glucosamine Sulfate Formula

Selection of the proper glucosamine product is essential if you wish to receive the same benefits demonstrated in the European clinical studies. Not all glucosamine products are created equal.

Historically, a number of different types of glucosamine have been tried with patients, with varying degrees of clinical success and complications. Some earlier glucosamine derivatives, for example, contained iodide ions. Precautions were required in patients with thyroid problems because of the small amount of iodide, which can be toxic.

Other glucosamine products, such as glucosamine hydrochloride (HCl), N-acetyl L-glucosamine, and glucosamine complex, have very little documentation and do not offer the same proven synergistic effect between glucosamine and sulfate. In the absence of therapeutic equivalence studies in patients, or at least of bioequivalence studies, any feature of efficacy or safety acquired on glucosamine sulfate cannot be transferred to other forms of glucosamine, because different salts of the same organic base may have totally different pharmacokinetic, efficacy or safety properties. Without the proof of bioequivalence with glucosamine sulfate, acetylated glucosamine or glucosamine HCL might not be bioavailable or effective; it could even produce a toxic effect. This is not a problem of *preference* but a fact, and the use of these other forms of glucosamine for osteoarthritis is not supported by adequate documentation at this time.

The highly active role of glucosamine in rebuilding cartilage is enhanced by its combination with sulfate, which in itself is another important component in the structure of proteoglycans. Moreover, sulfate is practically nontoxic, making it a much better choice than iodides.

Until recently, it was not possible to eliminate several unfavorable properties of the glucosamine sulfate compound, however, particularly its instability under normal background temperatures and humidity. Although injectable forms have long been available and have been well-studied clinically with extremely positive results, these are rather delicate to prepare and obviously are limited by their route of administration as to who can use them.

Delivery systems such as transdermal, nasal or transbuccal sprays have been developed for other products with transbuccal delivery demonstrating excellent absorption rates. These alternative delivery systems are likely to cost more, partly because their applications require extensive research and development in order to prevent the material breakdown of the substances that they are to deliver. However, they do show promise when these challenges are overcome, particularly for use with individuals who have digestive problems or who cannot swallow capsules.

In order to put glucosamine in capsule form, a manufacturing technique was required that would stabilize the material. In an entirely surprising discovery, it was found that it is possible to stabilize glucosamine sulfate by the formation of a mixed salt with sodium chloride. By combining glucosamine sulfate with the mixed salt and sodium chloride, the material's sensitivity to ambient relative humidity, even at high temperature, is practically negligible. In other words, the addition of mixed salts, including sodium chloride, stabilize the compound so that it may be kept at room temperature with normal levels of humidity without decomposing.

Rotta Research Laboratories of Milan, Italy developed this manufacturing process and holds the United States patent on the process for manufacturing the stabilized form of glucosamine sulfate. What's more, Rotta Research Laboratories has funded virtually all of the clinical trials. Rotta's is the only form of glucosamine to have been extensively clinically studied and proven to deliver the results discussed in this book.

To be sure, many other glucosamine sulfate products are available. It is reasonable to presume that they may work just as well, but so far specific studies on these products haven't been done.

In many cases, particularly in the nutritional industry where quality varies, it is extremely beneficial to consumers to use the same material as that which was used in clinical studies, especially when the manufacturing process itself is integral to the long-term stability and potency of the material used.

Through an exclusive international marketing agreement, it is now possible to obtain the actual substance supplied by Rotta Research Laboratories in the clinical trials—GS-500™ from Enzymatic Therapy of Green Bay, Wisconsin (see Resources).

This is the only product that we can strongly recommend at this time because it is the only substance conclusively proven to work in clinical trials.

## Bottom Line

Based on a thorough review of the pertinent literature, international experts have come up with the following guidelines to explain the benefits of glucosamine sulfate to you and your doctor.

1. Glucosamine sulfate is a medication for the basic treatment of osteoarthritis, relieving symptoms and having disease-modifying properties.
2. The symptomatic efficacy of glucosamine sulfate is comparable to NSAIDs.
3. Glucosamine sulfate has no noteworthy side effects (in contrast to NSAIDs).
4. After discontinuation of glucosamine sulfate, the beneficial effects continue for several weeks (in contrast to NSAIDs).
5. All joints can be treated with glucosamine sulfate. The clinical efficacy of glucosamine sulfate has been demonstrated in different locations of the body: hips, knees, fingers, spine.
6. All stages of osteoarthritis can be treated with glucosamine sulfate, even very late ones. Ideally, early osteoarthritis should be treated to stabilize cartilage metabolism and to normalize joint function.
7. Patients of all ages can be treated.
8. Glucosamine sulfate has a preventive and a therapeutic

effect on osteoarthritis and also on the damage from traumatic events.

9. The time for surgery can be temporarily postponed in case surgery is necessary. Glucosamine sulfate treatment supports the regeneration of the joint tissues and also the contralateral joints which are apt to be overused while the joints operated on are healing.

10. Glucosamine sulfate greatly improves the quality of life in patients with osteoarthritis.

# PART III

PART III

# 7
## Dietary Strategies for Managing Arthritis

*When Lydia, a 37-year-old woman with three children and a job as an order taker at a nutritional firm in Los Angeles, changed from a predominantly red-meat and dairy-based diet to one that was almost completely vegetarian with small amounts of safe seafood, her osteoarthritis greatly improved within a month.*

*At first, she complained about deprivation and she missed hamburgers, ice cream and other fatty foods, but over a short time, as Lydia began to see her new body emerging, lighter, more appealing, and much freer from pain and stress on her joints than ever before, she became a convert—a true believer in the power of healing foods. Today, the rewards of living pain-free are so great that Lydia could never go back to her old ways of eating.*

*Karen was a 40-year-old former actress and mother of two young children who loved to play the guitar. Her diet was a recipe for joint disaster. She was beginning to develop severe rheumatoid arthritis, and her doctor was suggesting the short-term use of powerful and potentially dangerous drugs such as methotrexate. Fearful of its side effects and of losing mobility, especially in her fingers, Karen visited a physician who practiced holistic or integrative healing practices. The first thing her physician asked of Karen was that she eliminate, at least temporarily, red meat and dairy from her diet, and that she start eating more seafood.*

*Within a month, Karen's swelling went down markedly, and her joint mobility increased, especially in her fingers. She even began playing her guitar again, and, while she felt rusty, her fingers felt freer than ever before to move up and down the fret board and pluck the strings. Karen also found, as she began taking better care of her health, that she could once again keep up with the activities of her two small children. The results were enough for Karen to stay with her new nutritional plan. The way she was feeling was largely due to her new passion for healthy, organic, fresh vegetables, fruits and whole grains and cutting down on unhealthy fats. "I'm convinced that sticking to my diet is key to my continued better health," she says. "That and playing music and spending more time with my husband. He's a lot happier too now that his cholesterol and blood pressure are both down, which is probably because of our improved diet. I served him grilled tofu with mushrooms, and he actually enjoyed the dinner. So did my son and daughter. I expected more resistance. It's great for all of us. My husband's losing weight; we're more active; we're committed to the program."*

We have found that when many of our patients eliminate red meat and dairy, their arthritic conditions also improve. This is the case whether they are suffering the terrible gritty pains of osteoarthritis or the burning inflammation of rheumatoid arthritis. Of course, dietary management for arthritis is a little more complex than simply eliminating red meat and dairy; indeed, removing these two foods doesn't always work for everyone and isn't always necessary. Other dietary strategies may prove even more useful. The message, however, is clear and worth emphasizing: diet works, and it works extremely well, especially for long-term healing and prevention.

Yet, in each clinical case, cause for improvement is different. Thus, the lesson we take from these two clinical histories is that similar diets may work, but for completely different reasons— and sometimes they work because of interrelated healthy influences stemming from one single dietary change. However, many different dietary approaches have been tried and used successfully for healing arthritis. In this chapter, we will present some of the more proven concepts.

Take Lydia's case. When Lydia began emphasizing more greens and other vegetables, fruits and whole grains in her family's daily meals, she began taking in much higher amounts of specific joint-healing vitamins and other nutrients, such as beta carotene, vitamin C, vitamin E, boron, copper and magnesium, in addition to numerous other as yet unidentified substances in these healthy foods.

Was this change in her nutrient mix the determining factor in the improvement in her disease? Or was the real key her loss of 15 pounds—or something completely different? With the dietary improvements, her husband's blood pressure dropped almost ten percent—and he became a much happier man. When husbands lighten up, play with the kids, act like normal human beings, wives' moods also tend to brighten. Perhaps her husband's improving health helped to cure Lydia by lightening her mood around the house. By helping more with their children, her husband helped to lift some of her burden and enabled her to feel free to undertake more healthy habits: diet, weight loss, exercise and stretching. Probably each of these diet-related outcomes, as disparate as they might seem at first, was a positive influence on the outcome of her disease and on her spirit, attitude and self-esteem.

In contrast, Karen was never overweight. Her rheumatoid arthritis was constantly aggravated by her fatty acid imbalance. Her diet of animal foods delivered too much arachidonic acid, which tended to act as a proinflammatory agent in her body. It was basically like dropping lighted matches into gasoline and then wondering why on earth a fire was erupting in her joints. Karen needed to put out the fire, but was fanning the flames of painful arthritis with her high saturated fat diet of beef and dairy. By cutting down on these proinflammatory foods and eating more seafood, which soothes the body's inflammatory pathways, Karen's body had the opportunity to turn on its own healing powers. We'll discuss these food-related arthritis triggers later on in this chapter, but the point we wish to make is that the mind-body connection is complex and doctors don't always know why certain healing pathways work.

We have many ideas, beliefs and theories to help explain the miracle healing powers of food, but not all of the answers. We know that sensible diets based on the principles discussed in this chapter can help people to lose weight, pack more nutrients into their diet, reduce exposure to toxins, hasten the body's elimination pathways, rebalance immune function and support healthy detoxification. Each of these benefits, and many others known and unknown, explain food's miracle healing powers. Each day we're finding out more about the power of foods. "We are what we eat" is something we learned from childhood. Eating right makes you feel right.

There are healing miracles of nature in food. We are certain that diet is absolutely critical to turning *on* the body's healing powers for reversing osteoarthritis and rheumatoid arthritis as well as many other maladies. Diet isn't the only answer, but for just about any condition, including optimal lifelong health, diet is a major part of the equation. When mishandled, diet can become a double-edged sword. Some people are caught in prisons of habitual destruction, causing their own arthritis or worsening their condition. We hope that this chapter will, if nothing else, stimulate *you* to make sweeping, revolutionary changes in your thinking about food. A sensible diet will improve your happiness, health, appearance, memory, sexual vitality and just about every aspect of your life. *Eat right. Be healthy.*

Knowing that diet has such a profound impact on their health will give new hope to arthritis sufferers. This chapter's important information can help you to gain new insights for improving the condition of your joints and your overall health. How important is diet statistically to healing arthritis? While no one has an exact figure, Dr. James C. Breneman, an expert in allergic arthritis, estimates in *Alternative Medicine: The Definitive Guide* that 60 to 80 percent of people would benefit from some type of dietary changes. From our experience, about *two-thirds* of patients greatly benefit from dietary changes of all kinds if for no other reason than their weight will stabilize at its optimal level.

Diet is especially important when it comes to long-term, chronic conditions such as early stage heart disease, borderline hypertension, mildly elevated cholesterol, adult onset diabetes, arthritis and even cancer prevention.

Two important voices on the impact of diet and nutrition on joint health are those of Seattle-based naturopaths and educators from Bastyr University, Michael Murray and Joseph Pizzorno. In their *Encyclopedia of Natural Medicine*, they write:

Diet has been strongly implicated in many forms of arthritis for many years, both in regards to cause and cure. Various practitioners have recommended all sorts of specific diets for arthritis. In general, since rheumatoid arthritis is not found in societies that eat a more "primitive" diet and is found at a relative high rate in societies consuming the so-called western diet, a generally healthy diet rich in whole foods, vegetables and fiber and low in sugar, meat, refined carbohydrate and saturated fat appears to be indicated in the prevention and possibly the treatment of RA.[42]

## The Weight Connection

When diet is combined with weight loss, the long-term benefits are probably the very best medicine of all. After all, the body's joints can stand only so much weight-bearing pressure. Getting body weight to an optimal level is extremely important. The joints get worn from carrying extra weight day in and day out. The effect is cumulative and takes its toll in the adult years when one day, a person's cushioning and joint integrity may simply fade away and disappear. If children are overweight when young, the odds are greater that they will suffer osteoarthritis as they approach middle age. Fortunately, many of our dietary recommendations, including eating more seafood and less fatty red meat and dairy, combined with exercise, will naturally help to optimize weight.

Can diet also help those who are already thin? *Yes*. Diet can help by eliminating allergens and triggers. Diet can also help by rebalancing the intake of inflammatory-related fatty acids and by making sure that there are more healthy oils and fats in the diet. These dietary bonuses work whether or not you are overweight because their effects are independent of reducing body mass.

Diet also works best when part of an entire holistic arthritis healing program including exercise and use of proper supplements as well as an emphasis on the mind-body connection.

## Diet Fundamentals

There's no getting around it. You need to seek quality in your diet. Emphasize fresh, organic fruits, vegetables, whole grains, legumes, nuts and seeds. Add some fish, particularly sea fish, such as tuna and salmon, which are high in beneficial omega-3 fatty acids. When you just can't turn down the meat, choose buffalo, range beef, rabbit, turkey or fresh game, such as vension or elk. If it's a choice between chicken or turkey, choose the turkey, which is lower in dangerous types of saturated fats that act as proinflammatories in the human body. If you must consume pork, choose the leaner cuts and avoid the use of nitrite additives whenever possible (nitrite is not only a common arthritis allergen, it can form carcinogenic nitrosamines). Fortunately, you can find nitrite-free pork at your local health food store.

## What about Fats?

Remember the old saying, "good cop, bad cop." Well, it's the same way with fats. By itself, fat is not bad. It's the type you ingest and the manner in which you accumulate it that causes trouble. The healthiest fats include olive, primrose, flaxseed and wheatgerm, as well as certain fish oils.

A diet with a wide variety of plant foods, enhanced with safe seafood and limited meat and dairy, is most apt to supply powerful healing vitamins and minerals, as well as substances known as phytochemicals or phytamins, which are neither vitamins nor minerals, but seem to have equal or, in some cases, greater healing power than these more well-known types of nutrients. Such diets are particularly rich in inflammatory-mediating omega-3 fatty acids, which may be especially helpful in cases of rheumatoid arthritis.

It's interesting that the expensive gourmet restaurants and the cheap drive-throughs have one striking similarity—high fat. You are probably better off with the supermarket salad bar or the fresh turkey from the deli counter.

Today, to counter the super high-fat American diet, too much emphasis is being put on *non*fat diets. Our bodies need fats. Indeed, fats are the primary materials for manufacturing our hormones. Fats are not the enemy *per se*. Just too much of certain types of fats—in particular, too much saturated fat found in red meat and in some dairy products is harmful.

Saturated fats are converted to arachidonic acid which is then incorporated into cell membranes and converted into prostaglandins, leukotrienes and thromboxane (PG-2, LKB-4 and A2 respectively), which cause inflammation.

However, other types of fats, such as those found in fish oils or flaxseed oil, divert the body's inflammatory processes into another direction. In this case a fatty acid called alpha-linolenic acid is converted to eicosapentaenoic acid (EPA) and docosahexaenoic (DHA) acid and finally into other prostaglandins, leukotrienes and thromboxanes called PGE-3, LKB5 and A-3. In the case of fish oils, the process is even more efficient. Unlike plant-derived oils, such as evening primrose and flaxseed, fish oils provide EPA and DHA directly to the body without requiring conversion. These are the good fats. These are also made part of cell membranes but they create prostaglandins that reduce the body's inflammation levels. To heal arthritis, it is essential to shift the body's production of potentially inflammatory prostaglandins and leukotrienes to those kinds that diminish inflammation. This can be done by emphasizing plant foods and certain fish and by avoiding or strictly limiting foods like beef, lamb, and dairy.

## What About Meat?

Should I eat meat? The answer is *Certainly not as much as you do now, if you're eating the typical American diet.*

In America and Canada, beef and poultry are the flesh foods of choice for most meat consumers. In primitive times, even our domestic animals foraged on a wide range of grasses, nuts and seeds. Today, modern beef cows are fattened up in their last few months by confinement into feed lots, curtailment of exercise and growth-stimulating hormone drugs that are put into in their feed and implanted in their bodies. As previously noted, modern beef supplies high amounts of saturated fat, causing a build-up of arachidonic acid in the body, which, in turn, stimulates the body's inflammatory pathways, aggravating rheumatoid arthritis. This same fatty acid imbalance is precipitated with frequent consumption of chicken and lamb, as well as high-fat dairy foods.

What's more, saturated fat-rich foods are calorie-rich, too. People who eat too many servings of meats like beef and poultry are frequently overweight; once again, this excessive weight puts added stress on joints. Overweight brings with it low self-esteem, which in turn is an added burden to the immune system.

We recommend that all arthritis sufferers rethink their diets on many levels. Some may realize that eating flesh foods does not reflect their values and they may choose to forgo these foods for moral and ethical reasons. Others may decide to eliminate or vastly reduce their intake of all flesh foods because they simply feel better. Still others may eat a semivegetarian diet. In this case, they may want to emphasize safe seafood as a protein source but rely mainly on plant-based foods. We'll talk more about both vegetarian and semivegetarian diets throughout this chapter and will give you important tips on which foods are the best for various types of arthritic conditions and which are the worst.

Tofu is an excellent meat substitute; it's rich in protein, magnesium and calcium and may also prove helpful in cancer prevention, especially for male and female reproductive cancers, and in lowering blood cholesterol.

## Dairy Foods and Arthritis

Dairy may be a *huge* culprit in worsening rheumatoid arthritis for a significant number of patients. From clinical experience, we have noted that when patients eliminate dairy from their diets, their inflammatory arthritis symptoms clear up—so much so that it seems almost miraculous. Our clinical findings are confirmed in published clinical reports.[43-45]

We sometimes recommend that RA patients eliminate *all* dairy for at least a week. This simple, quick test may bring surprising results which may be most important for women. You may want to try this test yourself. If your symptoms or condition improve, the culprit that is aggravating your arthritis could be either the saturated fat or perhaps some type of immune irritant or allergen, especially in cheese products.

*Connie, a 28-year-old television producer from San Diego, consumed a diet with generous amounts of dairy foods, especially cheese. Connie's doctor asked her to keep a journal in which she recorded everything she ate and the dates and times of her flare-ups. Two weeks of journal keeping showed that Connie's arthritis seemed to occur after certain types of meals, especially those that were highest in cheese and dairy.*

*Connie liked Mexican dishes traditionally slathered in queso or cheese. By eliminating such foods, Connie was able to completely stave off arthritis attacks for a month. However, when she ate another big cheese-rich dinner, her condition flared up, and her hands became swollen and immobile. Seeing results in such a plain cause-and-effect relationship stunned Connie. "I never realized diet could have such a huge influence on my health," she said. "No more dairy for me. I'm using easy-melt tofu cheeses with my Mexican dishes now and soymilk on my cereal. Most important: I'm almost completely free of any symptoms of arthritis."*

Connie's case is one of many that illustrates so clearly the amazing power of diet to help or hinder recovery from arthritis. In another case from the medical literature, arthritis expert Richard Panush, Chairman of the Department of Medicine at Saint Barnabas Medical Center in New Jersey, reports that a woman in her early 50s, was also extremely allergic to milk.[43] Indeed, when given unlabeled milk powder capsules that were equivalent to an eight-ounce glass of milk, she went into a full-out arthritic attack with swollen joints and extreme stiffness. The symptoms worsened within 48 hours of ingesting milk, but subsided thereafter. By keeping dairy products out of her diet, she so completely eliminated her arthritis that Dr. Panush published a paper on the topic. The results were confirmed when he was able to reproduce these same results in rabbits by switching their diet from water to milk, causing inflammation in their joints.[46]

There is also some evidence that people who are lactose intolerant, especially women, may be particularly susceptible to dairy-related arthritis. These people lack the enzyme lactase, necessary to digest milk sugar (lactose).

If dairy is a problem, you will find suitable substitutes at your health food store. "Milk" made with amazake, rice and soy all taste great on cereals. Soy cheeses work well for cooking many dishes. A word of culinary caution: some soy cheeses don't melt well at all, and some soy drinks don't work with coffee.

# Vegetarian Diets and Arthritis

Vegetarian diets are extremely helpful. They reduce the risk of heart disease, cancer and many other modern maladies and also seem to play a positive role in the outcome of arthritis cases. Several studies have looked at this relationship. In one study, 90 percent of people with arthritis who adopted a vegetarian diet enjoyed improved grip strength, less pain, joint swelling, tenderness and morning stiffness.[47] It is very exciting to note that striking improvements came within only one month.

The reduced intake of saturated fat in beef, lamb and dairy and elimination of various allergens such as gluten, refined sugar, strong spices and preservatives, probably helped as well. Weight loss, sometimes a beneficial bonus that comes with vegetarian diets, probably also helped. The greater nutritional density of the plant foods may have also helped.

## Food Allergies/Elimination Diet

Clinical experience has taught doctors that some foods are more likely to contain arthritis triggers than other foods. Elimination diets remove specific foods in order to detect hidden triggers.

Once again, we come back to beef and dairy, which seem to be two of the most common trigger foods.

Meats contain natural chemicals with the potential to act like antigens in the bodies of hypersensitive people. An antigen provokes an immune response which in turn causes the body to produce antibodies. These antibodies somehow end up attaching themselves to the antigens and other tissue materials and cellular debris forming circulating immune complexes that become embedded in the body's joint tissues, stimulating inflammation and subsequent joint deterioration. Some doctors call this "allergic arthritis" and treat it as a specific form of the overall disease.

Cured meats, such as bacon, hot dogs and cold cuts, contain

preservatives and other chemicals that are known to be more likely to trigger allergic arthritic symptoms in some patients.

People likely to suffer allergic reactions may suffer from what some practitioners call the "leaky gut" syndrome. In this condition, food or bacterial antigens pass into the bloodstream before they are completely digested by the stomach. It is also possible that bacteria in the gut may feed on particular foods and produce toxins. These then leak from the gut, and form circulating immune complexes, which attack the body's joints or cause an imbalance in the body's joint tissue-destroying enzymes such as collagenase, all of which result in further deterioration.

## Wheat, Corn and Cereals

Wheat and corn are also likely arthritis triggers. In one case, reported in the *British Medical Journal*, a woman suffered active rheumatoid arthritis for a quarter century without relief. Her drugs, the immune suppressant azothiaprin and aspirin, were not helping. Her physical health "was slowly but steadily going down," observed her doctor, Ronald Williams.[48] Medical sleuthing revealed that she had a corn allergy; unfortunately, corn was also being used as a filler in her medications. When she removed corn from her daily diet and changed medications, her symptom improvement within *one* week was "dramatic," according to Williams. Six weeks later, however, she relapsed. At first, the doctor thought that she had initially simply responded to the placebo effect of removing corn from her diet, *thinking* or *believing* that this would make a dramatic difference and thereby using the mind-body connection to actually think herself well. Alas, the mind-body connection was not the reason in this case. What happened was, unknown to her, she ate gravy made with corn flour. "She is now . . . feeling and looking better than she has done for over 10 years," says the doctor.[49]

In another case from our clinical experience, Linda came into the office extremely excited about her breakthrough discovery. She had eliminated wheat from her diet that week. "I've never felt better. I feel great. I can walk again without any hip problems." Within seven months, Linda was off hiking through the narrows of the Utah canyon lands.

Both wheat and corn are likely triggers for rheumatoid arthritis, and they are present everywhere in our diets. Both are used as main ingredients, additives and fillers not only in food products, but in over-the-counter and medical drugs. Be sure to read labels for all prepared and packaged foods, as well as OTC preparations and medical prescriptions.

Author Jean Carper offers this important report on cereals:

Italian investigators at the University of Verona tell of a patient who recovered from rheumatoid arthritis when she stopped eating cereals. Despite corticosteroid shots and oral gold salts, she got constantly worse until the physicians discovered that she had an allergic reaction to cereals. Consequently, they eliminated cereals from her diet for three weeks and she got dramatically better. As a test she again deliberately ate cereals, and her joint pain, morning stiffness and all other signs of rheumatoid arthritis returned. She banned cereal from her diet and the flare-ups stopped; she had no signs of arthritis for an entire year at the time of the report.[50]

## Nightshades

Could members of the nightshade family (tomatoes, eggplant, white potatoes and bell peppers) trigger arthritis? This theory stems from the work of Norman F. Childers, Ph.D., a University of Florida horticulture professor. Afflicted by a most severe crippling form of arthritis, Childers finally examined his diet in a last-ditch effort to heal himself. He discovered his attacks seemed to come hours after eating tomatoes. As a storehouse of plant lore, Childers knew that tomatoes were once thought to be poisonous. These members of the nightshade family contain the toxic chemical solanine.

By eliminating nightshades completely from his diet, Childers improved tremendously. Thousands of people have since written him attesting to their own recoveries after eliminating nightshades. No rigorous studies have ever been performed, but the professor estimates 10 percent of the population could be sensitive to the toxins in these plants.

From our own experience, we too have seen remarkable improvements in a limited number of patients who have removed nightshades from their diet.

Dr. Williams, whose patients have profited by removing food allergens such as corn from their diets, states:

> No one would be foolish enough to claim that every case of rheumatoid arthritis is associated with a food allergy, but if only one in 20 is—and I suspect that it is considerably more—I question whether we have the right to withhold such a simple, safe, brief and noninvasive investigation [of food allergy] in a disease of such appalling chronicity.[49]

We believe that the diet connection is essential in the overall evaluation of the arthritis patient. If your doctor won't work with you in examining your diet, find a health professional who will and who is informed about the arthritis-diet connection. We've listed a number of medical groups in the Resources section.

## Top 20 Rheumatoid Arthritis-Aggravating Foods

Based on the work of arthritis expert L. Gail Darlington, these are some of the worst foods for arthritis sufferers to consume.[51]

| Food | Percentage of People Adversely Affected |
|------|------------------------------------------|
| Corn | 56 |
| Wheat | 54 |
| Bacon/pork | 39 |
| Oranges | 39 |
| Milk | 37 |
| Oats | 37 |
| Rye | 34 |
| Eggs | 32 |
| Beef | 32 |
| Coffee | 32 |
| Malt | 27 |
| Cheese | 24 |
| Grapefruit | 24 |
| Tomato | 22 |
| Peanuts | 20 |
| Sugar | 20 |
| Butter | 17 |
| Lamb | 17 |
| Lemon | 17 |
| Soy | 17 |

# How to Do a Food Elimination Diet

According to both Lesley Houston and Amanda Ursell, writing in *The Practitioner*, the best method for investigating possible food intolerance to date has been by excluding all but a few minimal low-allergen foods from the diet for approximately two weeks. The safer foods are lamb, rice, carrots, cabbage, pears, high-oleic sunflower oil and seeds, filtered water and salt. If symptoms improve, other foods can be gradually reintroduced in a predetermined sequence to discover which foods produce symptoms in an individual patient. The culprits are then excluded from the diet.[52, 53]

Among the foods that Houston and Ursell find most likely to be associated with allergic arthritis are:

- Milk and dairy products
- Wheat, gluten and corn
- Beef
- Coffee
- Citrus fruits
- Tomatoes
- Peanuts

## Fasting

When done under proper supervision, fasting can also help in some cases of arthritis. No one is sure why. It may simply be that eliminating all foods removes the specific food triggers that were aggravating the condition. If foods are then returned to the diet singly and gradually, one can pinpoint arthritis trigger foods and avoid them in the future.

## Fish Oils and Arthritis

As mentioned earlier, certain seafoods rich in omega-3 fatty acids are extremely beneficial for anyone suffering from inflammatory types of arthritis, especially rheumatoid arthritis. Three or more servings weekly of select seafood dishes could do more for arthritis than any medical drug or surgery.

Salmon, tuna, sardines, herring, anchovies and mackerel are rich sources of omega-3 fatty acids, particularly two known specifically as docosahexaenoic acid (DHA) eicosapentaenoic acid (EPA). These fatty acids, found in such limited amounts in most people's diets today, suppress production of substances such as specific types of cytokines and leukotrienes that are produced by white blood cells and are responsible for the inflammation accompanying arthritis. Eating these healthy fats is likely to reduce the body's overall inflammation levels, thin the blood and reduce risk for heart attack and stroke, as well as arthritis.

*Three or more servings weekly of select seafood dishes could do more for arthritis than any medical drug or surgery.*

We've known for hundreds of years that fish oils play a role in arthritis. British doctors used to give their patients cod liver oil to alleviate rheumatism. Today, medical science has validated the importance of fish oils, especially for relieving rheumatoid arthritis.

In one study, researchers compared 324 rheumatoid arthritis cases with 1,245 controls.[54] They used a food frequency questionnaire to ascertain diet during a one-year period. Two or more servings per week of broiled or baked fish (but not of other types of fish) was associated with up to a 43-percent decreased risk of rheumatoid arthritis. These results support the hypothesis that omega-3 fatty acids may help prevent rheumatoid arthritis, and also that certain types of cooking, especially frying, destroy these types of fatty acids. More than six other extremely well-done studies confirm that certain fatty fish can help to dramatically curtail the suffering of inflammatory rheumatoid arthritis.[55] How much fish must one eat for an effect and for how long? Generally, about a seven- or eight-ounce salmon steak, two cans of sardines, or about three to four ounces of herring three to five times a week supply the necesssary amounts of DHA and EPA to make all the difference. Results may require a month to become apparent. Consuming these amounts of fish three to five days a week may be required to subdue active cases of rheumatoid and other inflammatory types of arthritis. For some people this may simply be too much seafood. For this reason, many medical experts recommend that persons with active arthritis, who are trying to suppress recurrences, consider taking fish oil capsules daily (see Chapter 9).

Indeed, our discovery, or rather rediscovery of this ancient healing secret, may hold the key to the safe healing of many patients with rheumatoid and other types of inflammatory arthritis. What's more, eating regular portions of these fatty fish may prevent arthritis entirely, as well as markedly reduce risk for heart disease.

## *Seafood Warning*

Unfortunately, some seafood is contaminated with chemical toxins which can increase risk for cancer and birth defects. The best sources of omega-3 fatty acids with the least contamination include rainbow trout from alpine lakes and streams, sardines, halibut, king salmon, tuna and sockeye. Stay away from any fish caught from industrialized inland waterways, as well as American eel and sablefish, which are contaminated. Tuna has low levels of mercury and could be toxic to the fetus of pregnant women. Tuna should be limited to once a week during pregnancy. Pregnant women should also use flaxseed oil rather than fish oil caps. Flaxseed oil works best when intake of other common cooking oils is sharply curtailed. Also, supplemental zinc may be required by the body to facilitate the conversion of alpha-linolenic acid (the omega-3 fatty acid constituent in flaxseed oil) to its fully formed cousins DHA and EPA. For a discussion of safe seafood, see *The Safe Shopper's Bible* by David Steinman and Samuel S. Epstein, M.D.

SAFEST SOURCES OF OMEGA-3 FATTY ACIDS IN SEAFOOD

Sockeye salmon
Albacore tuna
King salmon
Bluefin tuna
Pink salmon
Coho salmon
Anchovy
Atlantic salmon
Atlantic halibut
Sardines
Rainbow trout

# What about Cooking Oils?

We advise patients to avoid oils rich in common omega-6 type fatty acids, particularly corn, ordinary (nonoleic) safflower, sunflower and coconut and margarines made with hydrogenated oils. These oils can aggravate inflammatory arthritis, and also increase risk for heart disease. Instead, we recommend olive, walnut and high oleic sunflower and safflower oils. High oleic indicates those strains of safflower and sunflower that are high in monounsaturated fats. Flaxseed oil should not be heated.

Avoid deep frying foods, as frying damages cooking oils and causes oxidation. Once ingested, oxidized cooking oils stimulate the body to release harmful free radicals and proinflammatory histamines, leuokotrienes and cytokines which can burden the body's detoxification pathways. Also, frying produces carcinogenic substances in oils and destroys most of their fragile beneficial chemicals.

# A Shopper's Guide to Healthy Joint Foods

Many other foods, besides those thus far discussed in detail, are extremely important to cartilage, tendon, ligament and overall joint and skeletal health. We've presented these in an easy-to-use smart shopping chart. Look at all the wonderful foods you can purchase that supply so many great nutrients for your diet. Of course, if you are suffering from food-related allergies, some of these suggestions will be taboo for you. For most people, these are some of the very best foods for supporting health and for healing arthritis. Always choose organic whenever possible.

## Foods for Healthy Joints and Bones

| Food | Nutrient | Benefits |
| --- | --- | --- |
| Almonds, bok choy, broccoli, canned mackerel, salmon, and sardines (with bones), collards, filberts, kale, milk (low-fat, nonfat), okra, soy cheeses, tofu, turnip greens, yogurt (low-fat, nonfat) | Calcium | Vital to formation of strong, dense bones. Proven to slow bone loss in postmenopausal women. |
| Amaranth, artichokes, beet greens, black beans, broccoli, bulgur wheat, cereals, chard, dried apricots, dried beans, filberts, green vegetables, okra, peanut butter, seeds (pumpkin, squash, sunflower, water-melon), snails, spinach, swiss chard, tofu, wheat bran, wheat germ, white beans, whole wheat flour | Magnesium | More than half of all magnesium in the body is found in the bones. Many bone-building processes in the body involving calcium also depend on adequate intake of magnesium. |
| Kelp, leafy vegetables, fruits, nuts, whole grains | Boron | Improves calcium absorption and helps postmenopausal women maintain optimal levels of estrogen. Activates formation of vitamin D. |

| | | |
|---|---|---|
| Crabmeat, dark green leafy vegetables, dried beans and peas, lobster, nuts, oysters, vegetables (fresh), whole grain cereals and breads, yeast (dried) | Copper | Adequate amounts help prevent spontaneous bone fractures. Helps in formation of collagen for bone and connective tissue. Nearly 20 percent of body's copper is found in the skeleton, and a deficiency can result in bone demineralization. |
| Alfalfa, beets, bell peppers, brown rice, leafy green vegetables, rice bran, soybeans, unrefined whole grains | Silica | Necessary for bone and connective tissue formation, and calcium absorption. Contained in connective tissue and strengthens collagen. Necessary for maximum activity of several enzymes involved in bone and collagen synthesis. |
| Bran (unprocessed), Brazil nuts, crabmeat, dry beans, lentils, mussels, nonfat dry milk, oysters, pecans, peanut butter, pine nuts, seeds (pumpkin, sunflower, squash, and watermelon), spinach, squid, turkey (dark meat), wheat germ, whole grain cereals | Zinc | Necessary for collagen formation and for the body to use calcium. |

| | | |
|---|---|---|
| Fortified cereals, eggs, milk (vitamin D-fortified; low-fat nonfat), sunshine (stimulates body to produce vitamin D) | Vitamin D | Essential for the body to process calcium and phosphorous and is especially important for normal bone and tooth formation in children. |
| *Vitamin $B_6$*: Bananas, carrots, potato skin (boiled/baked), salmon (smoked), sauerkraut, spinach, tuna, turkey, watermelon *Vitamin $B_{12}$*: Abalone, anchovies, clams, crab, rabbit, salmon and sardines (canned), squid *Folic acid*: Artichokes, asparagus, beets, broccoli, bulgur, collards, mustard greens, okra, red kidney beans, spinach, turnip greens, white beans | Vitamins $B_6$, $B_{12}$, folic acid | Together, these three vitamins are able to reduce homocysteine concentrations in the blood; elevated levels of homocysteine are thought to play a role in osteoporosis by interfering with collagen cross-linking leading to a defective bone matrix. |
| Apple juice, blackberries, broccoli, Brussels sprouts, cantaloupe, cauliflower, cabbage, cherries, grapefruit juice, green and red peppers, guavas, kale, kiwi, oranges, papayas, peas, potatoes, strawberries, tangerines, tomatoes | Vitamin C | Essential for healthy collagen and connective tissue. Helps body utilize calcium. |

| Blackberries, blueberries, cherries, hawthorn berries, raspberries | Flavonoids | Helpful in stabilizing collagen, the major protein structure in bone. |
|---|---|---|
| Beans, miso, textured vegetable protein, tofu, tempeh, soymilk | Phyto-estrogens | High consumption correlated with low risk for osteoporosis and fewer menopausal symptoms; may also be helpful in an overall sense for arthritis by maintaining hormonal balance safely and effectively. |

## Diet and SLE

A low calorie, low fat diet may be of benefit to sufferers of lupus (SLE). It may be especially important to limit proteins with high amounts of the amino acids phenylalanine and tyrosine.[56] What's more, fish oils may also be extremely beneficial in preventing and reducing the severity of this disease.[57, 58]

## Diet and Gout

For gout, observe the following:

- Eat a diet low in purines (found in yeast extracts, offal, fish roe and herrings).
- Restrict alcohol intake.
- Moderate protein intake.
- Gradually lose weight.

## Diet and Ankylosing Spondylitis?

Interestingly, knowing something about the etiology of some cases of ankylosing spondylitis may provide some sketchy clues on diet. We know that some people with ankylosing spondylitis have a type of tissue that looks much like the *Klebsiella* bacteria normally living in the bowel. These bacteria feed on starchy carbohydrates and multiply, thus suggesting potential help for persons suffering from this condition by following these guidelines:

- Eat a low-carbohydrate/high protein diet.
- Reduce starchy foods, such as breads, pasta and potatoes.

## Keep a Food Diary

Keeping a journal can be a potent force for change, insight, spiritual growth and healing. We strongly advocate that you consider keeping one as you begin *Arthritis: The Doctors' Cure*. Such a journal should also be devoted to your daily food intake. Be sure to record all of the foods that you eat—every little topping, dressing and snack. Often, people grossly *underestimate* their daily calorie intake.

A good diet is inherently low in calories and contains the best fats. For nonpregnant and nonnursing women, however, if your diet is consistently about 1,500 to 2,000 calories, you're probably eating too much to lose weight—unless, of course, you're involved in physically demanding work or intensive exercise. For men, anything above 2,500 to 3,000 calories or more is a recipe for weight gain—again, unless, of course, you're involved in physically demanding work or intensive exercise, or are extremely large and active with a high metabolism. It isn't absolutely necessary to count calories if you're exercising three to five times a week and your diet is largely based on our recommendations; however, many excellent calorie-counting books are available which can help you to roughly estimate your calorie intake. Also record any flare-ups of your arthritis after certain foods or meals. This can provide tremendous insight. Keep your food diary for at least one month. The food diary is great vehicle for seeing the truth about your diet.

## Be Patient

You might not get there right away in terms of the perfect diet for your individual biochemical needs. We advise you to relax and enjoy the journey; try to focus on your goal of pain-free living.

For example, Connie made a thorough exploration of all of the new dairy substitutes that were available until she could find those that gave her some of the texture and taste of dairy without the hazards to her arthritis. She found certain brands of tofu cheeses worked extremely well on sandwiches, supplying much of the protein and calcium and other minerals of dairy without provoking arthritis attacks. Soy milk and *amazake* or rice milk tasted fine on her now organic cereals. By exploring her options and reaching a rational yet personal health decision, Connie was able to improve her condition a great deal—and without feeling too deprived.

In another case, Danielle, 37 and a well-known actress, could begin a low-fat diet with adequate control and avoidance of midnight munching when she stopped using various street drugs and replaced these addictions with healthy ones, such as running and aerobics. Only then did her body tell her it needed less of certain foods and more of others because she became attuned to her body.

In some cases, patients have returned to their old diets. They've begun consuming fatty foods such as chicken, cheese, beef, and coconut oils, all rich in specific inflammation-causing fats, and they've re-experienced joint swelling and morning stiffness.

Above all else, remember that food is as much a spiritual as it is biological necessity. Eating well means choosing foods for many reasons. Organic foods help to protect farm workers from pesticide exposures. Cutting down on hormonally-treated beef and dairy helps to end deplorable factory farming methods used for raising 99 percent of our livestock today. Food deserves our reverence. It in turn can unlock the healing powers within your body.

## Bottom Line

- Diet can help to reduce the symptoms of arthritis.
- Fats are not the enemy *per se*. Different types of fats have different types of effects on arthritis.
- Saturated fats promote the inflammatory process.
- Omega-3 fatty acids, on the other hand, calm down the inflammatory process and support immune function.
- Seafood and flaxseed oil provide beneficial omega-3 fatty acids.
- Elimination diets work; they can be used to identify food triggers.

· Weight reduction is beneficial for overweight patients with arthritis.
· A diet low in starchy foods may benefit patients with ankylosing spondylitis.
· Keeping a food diary can be extremely beneficial.

# 8
## Exercise

The least expensive, most productive, valuable health strategy now available is exercise. It's not complicated, it's cheap and you don't need special equipment. What's more, when you exercise, your body releases natural morphine-like substances called endorphins that imbue you with a wonderful sense of well-being. We're talking about good old-fashioned, perspiration-inducing, body-twisting exercise. Exercise is so important to your health that we can't say enough good things about it. And we can't stop talking about it or urging our patients to *do* it. Exercise is body talk. Exercise is health.

The funny thing is, most people, especially in the United States, exercise only enough to reach over and pick up the remote control or to make it to the bathroom during the half-time break of a National Football League game.

Exercise is important for much more than joint health. It vastly reduces the risk of heart disease, osteoporosis, diabetes, cancer and many other of our most notorious modern diseases. We know of one gentleman in his 80s who suffered a serious heart attack. It probably would have done him in if not for the fact that a lifetime of vigorous exercise, including handball, lacrosse and football, helped to build up collateral vessels leading to and from his heart. These collateral vessels helped him to keep a little blood flow moving through his body—enough to keep him alive long enough for the paramedics and then emergency room doctors to stabilize his condition, and, finally, to bring about his excellent recovery. Today, he is extremely active, again because of a lifetime of exercise.

Women can markedly reduce their risk of breast cancer with exercise, and exercise begun early enough can stave off the ravages of osteoporosis. Of course, exercise and diet combined are the best proven antidote to obesity. When you look good, you feel good, and that does wonders for your self-esteem and resistance to disease.

Although regular physical activity is associated with important physical and mental health benefits, an estimated 53 million U.S. adults are inactive during their leisure time. While Americans on the whole do not exercise enough, persons with arthritis and other rheumatic conditions are the worst offenders; yet, the very activities that they avoid are ones that could actually help them to feel better.[59]

What is exercise? Exercise can be better understood when we examine what we expect as the end result: Some exercises, such as weight lifting, are designed to primarily improve muscle size and strength. Other exercises, such as stretches and yoga, are adept at improving flexibility and keeping the body limber. Still other exercises, such as hiking and running, increase endurance. Of course, one particular exercise may fulfill each of these mandates to different degrees.

"We have 30 acres on this side of the highway that we walk around, sometimes with the dog, sometimes with my son Shelby. I also do gardening, which some people don't think of as exercise, but it sure does the trick," country singing star Reba McEntire says, referring to how she maintains her great looks and energetic lifestyle.

Meanwhile, yoga, one of Courtney Cox's exercises of choice, helps to "tone and elongate every muscle in the body." Exercising "has helped my posture a lot, which I think is very important to good health," she adds.

Golf. Biking. Tai chi. Yoga. Walking. Tennis. Gardening. Sit-ups. Push-ups. Aerobic dance. Swimming. The point is, to get started. Exercise is one of the most powerful healing tools available to you. No matter what your age, the scientific evidence is in: Some form of exercise is always beneficial to your health.

Every time you exercise, you put pressure on your joints. Because joints have no blood vessels, they rely on the exchange of fluids through the membranes in order to eliminate toxins and receive nutrients. Every time you exercise you cause this nutrient and toxin exchange process. Your joints receive more nutrition. This then stimulates cell regeneration processes. Exercise also strengthens muscles, bones, tendons and ligaments, which are integral to your overall structural health and can help to compensate for weakened joints.

### How Exercise Helps

- Strengthens muscles, bones, tendons and ligaments, which compensates for weakened joints.
- Flushes fluids in cartilage, bringing nutrients in, toxins out.
- Stimulates healthy cell division and regeneration.
- Limbers and tones entire body.

## Exercise and Arthritis

Until recently, the conventional wisdom among doctors was that inflamed joints required rest. Gradually, however, doctors advanced their thinking to the point where they concluded that exercise probably would not hurt, and even might help in some cases, but that it could not be universally recommended for relieving symptoms or maintaining or increasing joint function.

The fact is, exercise does help. It doesn't hurt. We're proexercise. For one, we've always known that the arthritis sufferer tends to engage in less leisure time activity than nonsufferers. As a result, their risk for other diseases such as heart disease, obesity, osteoporosis and diabetes is likely to increase. Therefore, if for no other reason, exercise is important to reduce the risk of these other serious killer diseases. However, clinically, we've seen many patients who exercise improve greatly, to the point where they can reduce their medication or forgo it altogether. Finally, the most recent studies on exercise and arthritis have presented strong evidence that exercise really does help.[60] It may not be a cure-all and it may not take the place of glucosamine sulfate, but exercise is extremely important.

In a sense, then, we are witnessing a thoughtful reevaluation of physical exercise as a therapeutic modality for arthritis patients—despite earlier concerns that exercise might exacerbate joint symptoms or accelerate disease.[61]


## Sampling the Studies

In 1997 a study was published to examine the effectiveness of a group exercise program for 40 patients with osteoarthritis of the knee who had been referred for physiotherapy.[62] The study, carried out in the outpatient department of a large public hospital, was based on repeated measures with a two-month follow-up. On completion of the program more than 90 percent of the 40 patients showed significant improvements in pain and performance without increases in medication, use of walking aids or fatigue. The gait variables of velocity, cadence and stride length demonstrated significant increases. All improvements were maintained at the two month follow-up assessments. This study suggests that exercise can indeed reduce pain and increase physical function in persons with osteoarthritis of the knee.

In another study published in the same journal and also on persons with osteoarthritis of the knee, patients in the treatment group experienced a feeling of overall improvement in the knee, and their ability to descend steps improved when compared to the control group.[63]

Exercise also helps rheumatoid arthritis patients. In one study published in 1997 in the *Journal of Rheumatology*, the effect of resistance exercise was studied in patients with fairly advanced stages of rheumatoid arthritis.[64] Forty-nine rheumatoid arthritis patients, 37 women and 12 men between the ages of 35 and 76, with an average age of about 61, were randomly assigned to exercise and control groups for a 12-week resistance muscle-training program. A circuit weight-bearing form of training was incorporated, using light loads with high repetitions. A videotape demonstrating the exercises was given to all exercising participants to enable them to continue the program at home at least three times per week. A significant improvement at 12 weeks was noted in the exercise group for self-reported joint count, number of painful joints, sit-to-stand time, grip strength, knee extension and dexterity.

In 1997 yet another report, this one published in *Research in Nursing and Health*, confirmed the great help that exercise provides for rheumatoid arthritis patients.[65] The effects of 12 weeks of low-impact aerobic exercise on fatigue, aerobic fitness and disease activity were examined in 25 adults with rheumatoid arthritis. People who participated more frequently reported decreased fatigue, while those who participated less frequently reported an increase in fatigue. All subjects, on average, showed increased aerobic fitness and increased right and left hand grip strength, decreased pain, and decreased walk time.

Dancing and water aerobics are also great exercises for persons with rheumatoid arthritis.[66, 67]

The effects of physical training on elderly fragile patients with rheumatoid arthritis on low-dose steroids were also investigated to make sure that there was no upper age limit.[68] The controlled study included 24 patients who had been treated with low-dose steroids for two years. Each patient was assigned either to a treatment group receiving training or to a control group not receiving training. The training took place over a three-month period and was based on a protocol using progressive interval training consisting of bicycle exercises, heel lifts and step-climbing. The exercises were performed twice weekly for 45 minutes. Comparison of the two groups showed that disease activity did not increase in the trained group and that fewer swollen joints were observed in this group. The work capacity of the trained patients was doubled, and the numbers of repetitions increased 76 percent. The researchers concluded that individually adapted exercise programs can be recommended for elderly rheumatoid arthritis patients on steroid treatment.

In a 1994 study in the *Scandinavian Journal of Rheumatology*, 39 consecutive patients with recent-onset rheumatoid or other forms of arthritis were randomly assigned either to a strength-training group or nonexercise group for a six-month period.[69] During the study period significant improvements took place in the exercise group in maximal muscle strength for all examined muscle groups as well as in red blood cell sedimentation rate. Erosive changes in joints increased much less in the exercisers than in the nonexercisers.

For elderly patients, we add this note of caution: Years of inactivity may have reduced your cardiovascular health so much so that you should work with your health professional to create an

exercise program that stays within your current physical limitations. Remember to go slow, but be steady and consistent. Also,
if you suffer muscle soreness, be sure to use combination enzymes
for safely reducing pain and inflammation (see Chapter 9).

## Stretching

Stretching is one of the best exercises for people with arthritis
and those who wish to minimize their risk for arthritis later on in
life. Stretching helps to keep bodies limber and vital and fights
premature aging. Stretching improves circulation *and* mental
attitude.

Stretching involves two types of movements: range-of-motion
and isometric. Range-of-motion exercises emphasize movement.
Isometric exercises use an opposing force, yet also do well for
stretching and limbering muscles and joints. Range-of-motion
movements are always done *before* isometric exercises.

We recommend that everybody who wishes to maximize their
health stretch for 30 minutes at least three times a week in addition
to regularly doing strength, agility and endurance exercises.

### STRETCHING TIPS

- If your joints hurt, try an exercise or movement that is less
  painful. Do not try to forcibly work through your joint
  pain.
- Work slowly and steadily.
- Try holding the movement at the point you feel a
  comfortable stretching sensation in your joints. Each
  movement should be done until you feel your muscles and
  joints have been adequately stretched and toned.

- Even though an exercise is usually named for the specific body part that it primarily stretches, it probably will exercise and stretch other body parts as well. Try to think of each movement as a whole body stretch, emphasizing one particular joint area. Shoulder shrugs, for example, also may help the lower back and calves if done as full body stretches.
- For any exercise, if you feel pain or dizziness, stop and talk to your doctor.

We recommend the basic stretches below. Work up to about 25 repetitions for each movement.

## Neck Stretches

**Chin-to-chest flex** firms and tones muscles of neck, cranium and shoulders, loosens up vertebrae and trapezoid muscles. Neck flexing can even help to avoid a facelift by strengthening sagging neck and chin muscles. This movement is especially beneficial for people who are desk-bound, especially if they work at a computer keyboard.

*How to do:* Touch chin to chest. Then raise chin to point to ceiling or sky cradling your head in your hands to protect your neck. Repeat. Work up to 25 repetitions.

**Shoulder to shoulder stretch** loosens the muscles on the side of the neck.

*How to do:* Stretch neck from one shoulder to the other. Repeat. Work up to 25 repetitions.

**Eye to sky stretch** supports healthy joints and muscles throughout the cranium.

*How to do:* Stand straight. Bend your head as far back as it can comfortably go, cradling your head in your hands. Feel muscles throughout neck and head working. Return to upright position. Work up to 25 repetitions.

**Hand against side of head (isometric)** strengthens and firms up neck muscles.

*How to do:* Put hand against left side of head and push with neck while resisting with hand. Repeat on right side. Hold six seconds. Work slowly up to 25 repetitions.

**Hand against forehead (isometric)** strengthens and firms muscles in back of neck.

*How to do:* Put hand against forehead. Try to push forehead down while resisting. Hold six seconds. Work slowly up to 25 repetitions.

**Hand against back of head (isometric)** strengthens and firms front neck muscles and joints and muscles of chin.

*How to do:* Put hand or hands against back of head. Try to look up while resisting the motion. Hold six seconds. Work slowly up to 25 repetitions. Repeat with other hand if working with just one hand.


## Shoulder Stretches

**Arm and shoulder rotation** helps to keep the deltoids flexible. This movement also helps to keep arms and fingers flexible, as the stretching proceeds from the fingertips all the way to the deltoid.

*How to do:* Rotate arms in circles with a gradually widening radius. Work up to 25 repetitions.

**Shoulder shrug** helps to maintain good solid posture and can even help the lower back and calves if done with full-body stretching.

*How to do:* Lift shoulders up and rotate, first in one direction, then in the other. You'll feel your chest and calf muscles stretch, too. That means your whole body is part of the stretch. Work up to 25 repetitions.

**Arm raise** helps to prevent compressed spine, besides loosening up the shoulder muscles.

*How to do:* Hold arm straight out extended fully in front of your chest. Raise to sky and really str--etch to the ceiling! Work up to 25 repetitions.

**Elbow touch** helps to stretch the tendons and ligaments and firm the muscles on the back of the arms and across the chest. It also helps the side muscles all the way up to the ears.

*How to do:* Clasp hands behind back of head. Try to touch elbows in front of body (around face) and then come back to starting position. Work up to 25 repetitions.

## Hip Exercises

**Knee to chest touch** helps to limber up the hips, lower back and knees.

*How to do:* Do when waking in the morning in bed or on the floor. Lift both knees at once and touch them to your chest, holding for five seconds, using your hands. Get on the floor and roll on your back forward and backward and side to side. Work up to 25 repetitions.

**Back thigh lift** is extremely important for strengthening the lower back muscles. An isometric exercise, it will also help to tighten the buttocks. People may feel some cramping the first few times they do this exercise. However, over time, the movement offers excellent protection against lower back problems.

*How to do:* Lay on your stomach. Try lifting your thigh off the floor, as high as possible, keeping your leg straight. Be sure to keep your hips on the floor. Alternate each thigh. Work up to about 15 repetitions.

## Knee Exercises

**Knee-calf tensor** is one of the most important physical therapy exercises that people with osteoarthritis of the knee can do. It helps to stabilize the knee and stretch out the leg muscles.

*How to do:* While sitting in a chair, rest your legs (one at a time) on a second chair or table. Extend your leg out as straight as possible. Point your toes toward your chest, really feeling the muscles of the legs being stretched. Work up to 10 to 15 repetitions.

## Leg Stretches

**Leg raises** are the basic strengthening movement for the quadriceps, the major frontal thigh muscle group. Another benefit to be derived from leg raises is that they are excellent for slimming the belly and strengthening the abdominal muscles, as well as strengthening the legs in general.

*How to do:* While on your back, raise one leg, keeping it straight, as high as you can. Be sure to keep your back on the floor and hold your legs in this position for five seconds. After holding the position, bend the leg at the knee and stretch some more, touching your knee and thigh to your abdomen.

## Back Exercises

**Abdominal raises** strenghten the abdominal muscles which in turn support the back.

*How to do:* While on your back, bend your knees. Raise your head with your arms straight out, touching your knees. Hold this position for five seconds. Work up to 15 repetitions.

**Back Extender** helps to loosen up the back.

*How to do:* Put your hands against a solid wall or pole and push your back in toward the wall or pole, letting all the muscles of your back stretch out. Work up to 25 repetitions.

### Chest Exercises

**Back flying motion** helps both the chest and back.

*How to do:* While standing, lift your arms to shoulder height and stretch back behind you, like a bird in flight. Work up to 25 repetitions.

## Conditioning and Strengthening Exercises

Some exercises are meant to increase the pumping power of the heart and strengthen the cardiovascular system. Examples of these include light to heavy weight-lifting, tennis, soccer, baseball, softball, basketball and touch football. Playing basketball, softball or soccer are other good forms of stretching-type exercises that will definitely limber and tone up the body. Many of the traditional Chinese movement exercises like tai chi and chi gong ho, which emphasize total balance and relaxation, are also excellent.

Cross-training is important. Vary your exercises. Walkers, for example, should also address their abdominal and upper body areas. Walkers need to do a lot of stretching because walking tends to use the same muscles over and over. Bicyclists need to do trunk-twisting exercises. Golf and tennis stretch one area of the body more than the other, so players should be sure to exercise the neglected side. For example, golfers should do some exercises for the lower body, as well as weight-bearing exercises. Cross-training can maximize the benefits of exercise for those with osteoarthritis by allowing the body to intuitively take advantage of stretching, strength training and aerobic exercise.

## Aerobics

Aerobic exercising, which involves jumping, trunk twisting and other athletic movements, not only builds strength and endurance but is also an excellent method for stretching the entire body. In low-impact aerobics, one foot always remains on the floor. In high-impact aerobics, both feet may leave the floor. Very likely, low impact aerobics will be appropriate for persons with osteoarthritis, especially of the hips or knees.

## Bicycling

Bicycling for endurance and strength is especially helpful and better than running for people with arthritis because the joints do not receive the pounding that occurs with running. Bicycling can be extremely beneficial but may not promote full flexibility because the bicyclist's posture remains static over extended periods of time. For this reason, bicyclists should be sure to stretch before and after their exercise. Bicycling may also irritate the prostate, so be careful, but by all means enjoy your cycling treks on trails, asphalt, other roads and off the road. Some types of bicycling, like trail riding, actually do exercise much of the body because of all of the twisting and dodging required to avoid rocks and other obstacles in the trail. Be sure, however, to wear protective gear, including a helmet and, possibly, knee and elbow pads.

## Chi Gong Ho

Chi gong ho was popularized by Bill Moyers in his TV special *Healing and the Mind*. This series of breathing and movement exercises is based on ancient Chinese principles of self-healing. Its meaning is taken from the Chinese *chi* for energy and *gong* for cultivation. Chi gong ho has been proven over time to be extremely helpful in reducing joint pain and enhancing mobility. *Chi* is a powerful energy force that, in Chinese medicine, is thought to nourish all of the muscles and organs. The exercises and movements, which can be learnt at local colleges, YMCAs and other learning centers, help to stimulate chi that flows throughout the body.

## Dancing

Don't neglect dancing as a form of exercise. Some square dancers may cover as much as five miles a night. Dancing is a great exercise for strength, stretching and endurance. Dancing can also help to bring couples together emotionally, spiritually and romantically.

## Golf

Golf enhances upper body movement while placing minimal strain on the knees and joints. If you are suffering severe osteoarthritis, however, you might want to ride in a cart rather than carry your clubs. Otherwise, use a pull cart and enjoy the cardiovascular workout for a full 18 holes.

## Hiking

An all-around great exercise for strength, endurance and stretching, hiking is also an enriching spiritual experience. Placing one's self in nature usually produces harmony of thought and a more relaxed state. Deepak Chopra advises half an hour to an hour daily in nature, appreciating its harmony and elegance. We agree. Hiking is a great way to prevent osteoarthritis; however, if you already have arthritis, you may have a difficult time going downhill for long periods and find that your knees hurt. Be sure to know your limitations and plan accordingly.

## Jumping Rope

A great stretching and endurance exercise, jumping rope can be done by people of all ages. A jump rope is an excellent exercise tool for travelers, because it is so light to carry. Jumping rope is also a great calorie burner and promotes nerve connections between all parts of the body and the brain, quickening reflexes. If your joints are extremely swollen or painful, however, this high-impact activity may not be best for *you*.

## Karate

Training in karate or in the other martial arts is a great overall way of stretching all of your muscles, as well as improving self-confidence and self-esteem. Women can especially benefit from karate and the other martial arts.

## Knitting

For improving joint mobility, especially for the fingers and wrists, knitting can be extremely helpful.

## Playing a Musical Instrument

Strictly speaking, playing music may not be an exercise, but it is excellent for improving joint mobility, especially in the fingers. We recommend playing musical instruments, especially for rheumatoid arthritis sufferers, as this form of exercise can help to keep the fingers and other joints of the hands and wrists flexible.

## Running

Running is a great endurance builder. The pounding the joints take may require that you run on grass or on a running track, use high-quality running shoes or both. Some people may find running exacerbates their arthritis. Shorter strides can minimize the impact on joints. A lot of people are enjoying mountain trail running, which provides high stress on the ankles. Be sure your ankles are ready for the trail before just taking off.

## Stair Climbing

The equivalent of running, stair climbers get as good a workout in 12 minutes as runners do in 20 minutes. Stair climbing helps to exercise the back, buttocks and lower legs. However, stair climbing is not advised for people with osteoarthritis of the knees.

## Tai Chi

Another ancient Chinese movement exercise, tai chi takes the student through a series of movements done with grace, concentration and focus, mimicking movements of daily life. This exercise may offer extremely important benefits to persons with arthritis, especially osteoarthritis. It is a great stress buster, too.

## Tennis

Although excellent for the heart and for limbering up the muscles, people with severe lower body joint problems of the ankles, knees, hips or spine may find the harsh pounding of tennis too much.

## Walking

Most people can enjoy the benefits of walking, either outdoors or on electric treadmills, although some may find walking makes their knees, hips, ankles or feet too sore. Adjust your personal walking program accordingly.

## Water Exercises

We also recommend exercise with water calisthenics, especially for those with arthritis. Almost anyone can enjoy the benefits of aerobic exercising in water. By using a water vest or life jacket, one can go beyond swimming laps and actually do a number of stretches and movements which on dry land might involve too much pounding. The buoyant water removes any load on the joints. You can lay in the water and kick your feet or just wade in the water for excellent resistance exercise. Wading back and forth in four feet of water can even help heal some osteoporotic bone fractures. As bone strength and joint health increase, one can slowly increase the intensity of the exercise.

## Weight-bearing Exercises

One of the overall best activities for those with arthritis is weight-bearing exercise. People whose bones have been weakened by osteoporosis, however, must begin an easy and safe exercise program under medical supervision. Even a slight stress on fragile bones could result in fracture. If you choose weight-bearing exercise, start with extremely light amounts of resistance. If possible and safe, high-intensity strength or resistance training is best.

## Yoga

Excellent for increasing range of motion, cardiovascular health and even strength, yoga is also excellent for reducing stress. It is a great stretching form of exercise. Yoga also has a spiritual component and can enhance your mood and attitude.

## More Exercise Benefits

Quite apart from its ability to reduce the risk of many other diseases, including heart disease, cancer and diabetes, exercise also has other important health benefits.

Researchers from the University of Nebraska have found that exercise such as jogging on a treadmill can boost testosterone levels by 30 percent. This in turn stimulates muscle growth and building.

For women at all stages of life, exercise is essential to skeletal health. That women of all ages need exercise is as true for daughters as for mothers and grandmothers. University of North Carolina researchers recently reported, for example, that very active female college freshmen who also had a high calcium intake had nearly 17 percent more bone density than their less active peers with lower calcium intake. Furthermore, freshmen who exercised at least four hours a week had even stronger bones; the amount of calcium they consumed was less important.[70]

In the December 28, 1994 *Journal of the American Medical Association*, Tufts University and Pennsylvana State University researchers reported on the impact of high-intensity strength training on 40 postmenopausal women whose ages ranged from 50 to 70 years of age; none of these women were using estrogen, exercised regularly, or were suffering osteoporosis. The women were divided into groups. One group, using pneumatic exercise machines for 45 minutes, two days a week for a year, exercised to strengthen their hips, knees, back and abdomen. The other group did not exercise.

One year later, the women who were engaged in the high-intensity exercises exhibited an increase in bone density in the area of their hips and spine. This is an important finding, as these areas of women's bodies are most vulnerable to osteoporosis-related fractures and osteoarthritis. The women who did not exercise suffered loss of bone density. The women who exercised also demonstrated increases in muscle mass, muscle strength and balance; these improvements help prevent falls in older women. In this sense, the study demonstrated that exercise may be even more effective than estrogen. While estrogen will help women retain bone density, exercise not only builds bone density but increases muscle mass, strength and balance; estrogen does not affect any of these areas. This is all helpful to the arthritis sufferer. Healthy muscles, bones, tendons and ligaments can compensate for some joint damage.

In another study, Dr. Steven Lindheim of the University of Southern California School of Medicine and coinvestigators found that even moderate exercise (30 minutes of aerobic activity three times a week) among postmenopausal women confers protection against cardiovascular disease. "The findings underscore the importance of physical fitness and its potential benefits to women who do not wish to take estrogen but still want to protect themselves against cardiovascular disease," said Lindheim.[71]

\* \* \*

Aerobics, swimming, walking, kick boxing, jump roping, jogging, hiking, walking. Do it all while you can. Any way you desire.

GOLDEN RULES OF EXERCISING

Whether your exercise is low-impact aerobics, tennis, light weight resistance, rapid walking, jogging, hiking, or even pool activity, the point is to exercise consistently three to four times weekly for at least three to four hours total duration, or about an hour to 90 minutes per session. Start easy. Build up your endurance, gradually exercising for longer periods until you reach an hour or longer. You will receive an enormous health dividend. Your body will feel better. Your mind will feel better. You'll live longer.

Listen to your body. Don't make your joints go places they really don't want to go. For example, not everyone can assume the lotus position in yoga. Even sitting cross-legged may be physically difficult for some people.

## Keep an Exercise Diary

As with diet, it is helpful to keep an exercise diary. Express your feelings. Are you feeling great or not so good? Enthused or bored? How can you motivate yourself to keep on exercising? You might want to make your exercise diary part of an overall healing journey journal as described in Chapter 10.

## Glucosamine Sulfate—Sports Medicine of Choice for Weekend Warriors and Professional Athletes

In more than 20 international clinical trials involving some 6,000 patients, glucosamine sulfate has been proven to dramatically reduce the pain and severity of osteoarthritic conditions. Now glucosamine sulfate, so successfully used among weekend athletes and others who are suffering from the debilitating ravages of osteoarthritis, is being used intensively by elite athletes for healing and prevention of sports injuries.

"I would say anywhere from 30 to 50 percent of our players are using glucosamine sulfate," says Kent Johnston, strength and conditioning coach of the 1997 Super Bowl Champion Green

Bay Packers. He adds that trainers from other professional sports teams in the National Football League and National Basketball Association have also begun providing their athletes with glucosamine sulfate.

"In the past, we've been very concerned with building men and women muscularly and strengthening them. However we've kind of left out the fact that those muscles are joined together by various connective tissues. Now we recognize that strengthening our players' joint matrix—cartilage, ligaments and tendons—is crucial."

Certainly, glucosamine sulfate cannot prevent every injury to a professional athlete; however, studies have shown that athletes and performers, such as football players and dancers as well as high school athletes, are at higher risk for osteoarthritis. Nevertheless, says Johnston, "the hitting, the ferocious contact that takes place not only in practice but on the field, really takes its toll, so as the season wears on in any sport, a product like glucosamine sulfate becomes even more important."

## The Bottom Line

- Exercise at least three to five times a week for at least an hour or longer.
- If you are suffering from severe arthritis, heart disease or other health problems, work with your doctor or health care professional to develop an exercise program that gradually increases in intensity. It is important to pace yourself and never exceed your sense of physical comfort. A little physical discomfort is all right as long as it is still within your capabilities, but don't go beyond what is uncomfortable or you could do long-term injury. Remember, it is better to

go out every day than go out hard once a week and quickly burn out.

- Stretch three to five times a week for at least 30 minutes a day.
- Above all else, be patient. If you don't exercise one day, remember there is always another chance tomorrow to be your best. Don't go too fast and burn yourself out after a few days. The object is to keep exercising for the *rest of your life*.

# 9

# Other Nutritional Supplements

Dietary supplements cannot take the place of good health habits, but they can help to make up for poor health habits. Indeed, they seem to work best when one's lifestyle habits or nutritional needs are at their worst. Malnourished children tend to benefit more from nutrients than marginally nourished children, as one example. No nutritional supplement has been clinically proven to heal osteoarthritis to the extent to which glucosamine sulfate has. None even comes close in terms of medical validation. Fish oils and oral enzymes are well-proven, but they work primarily only for rheumatoid and other inflammatory forms of arthritis. As for the rest of the nutritional supplements we'll discuss in this chapter, most do have direct human or anecdotal evidence, and almost all have experimental evidence; only a few have only an underlying theory of why they may be helpful.

The trend toward the use of nutrients in medicine perhaps owes much of its modern impetus to the seminal work of Janet Travell and David Simons, *Myofascial Pain and Dysfunction: A Trigger Point Manual*, published in 1983, which became and remains the most widely sold medical text worldwide. This book not only addresses the identification and treatment of dysfunctional myofascial (muscle/connective tissue) illnesses, but also discusses nutritional deficiencies.

Intrinsic in the work of Travell and Simons is the recognition of deficiency and perpetuating factors. The heaviest attention is paid to the water-soluble vitamins—particularly vitamin C and various B vitamins such as thiamine (B-1), riboflavin (B-2), panthenol (B-5), pyridoxine (B-6), hydroxycobalamin (B-12) and folic acid. The role of vitamin C is particularly supportive directly and indirectly in its antioxidant capacity and its role in healing when myofascial pain states are associated with various chronic illnesses such as viral syndromes.

Much of this information is not new. Although popularized by Drs. Travell and Simons, it has fortified the medical literature since the early 1950s, having been widely published in prestigious publications such as the *Journal of the American Medical Association.*

Today medicinal herbs are also attracting considerable attention for pain relief of inflammatory and other degenerative conditions, including osteoarthritis and rheumatoid arthritis. The profitability of their manufacturing and sales is causing an herbal boom, as consumers are becoming more actively involved in self-treatment. The general areas that herbs address include pain, fatigue, sexual well-being, appetite, sleep, mood and concentration. While there are sporadic claims of increased longevity and either the prevention or elimination of cancer, most benefits are in the area of "sense of well-being"—especially pain relief.

There is a strong historic basis for many of these claims, extending well back into the natural health literature and the general practices of many indigenous cultures. In the Southwest, particularly, the Indian heritage is rich with medicinal herbs, and there is an increasing respect for traditional Chinese medicine in the western world. Indeed, integrative medicine often makes use of Asian herbal remedies knowing that they are from a system that is over 5,000 years old.

The use of herbs, minerals and vitamins to relieve inflammation and for various pain states is thus playing an increasingly vital role. The data surrounding these substances is increasingly easy to obtain through the Internet, and various trusted authoritative publications available at better newsstands, health food stores and book stores.

However, it is important to recognize that pain states may have different etiologies and perpetuating factors. Your pain may be different than your friend's pain, and what works for you may not work for him or her and vice versa. Most important is a fair understanding of the diagnosis and how its pathophysiology came to bring about the dysfunctional state that's causing pain. This requires some reasonable medical knowledge and frequently some testing. All substances discussed in this chapter have both a therapeutic and possibly, in some cases, a toxic profile. While the risk/benefit profile on many of these substances is excellent, the suggestion of using multiple substances in combination should best be designed by a health professional. In addition, these therapies should be coupled with a general awareness in health and exercise, and a general avoidance of pollutants or factors in the environment that tend to offset the beneficial effects of many of these products. It is also best to work with a company that has a wide variety of products that are rigorously controlled for standards of purity. The company should have people available by phone to help explain the use of their products. Patients must actively participate in their health care by becoming knowledgeable and following through on reasonably designed regimens. This should be in cooperation with their health care advisors and continue to be monitored on a regular basis.

With these thoughts in mind, the popularity of vitamins, minerals and herbs is deserved and, as such, should be included in the quest for staying healthy.

This is especially important for people with arthritis. Many people simply have lived unhealthy lives by the time they visit their doctor. What's more, arthritis patients are likely to suffer malnutrition and have extensive nutritional needs that may not be completely addressed by the American diet. Some studies indicate that 50 to 75 percent of arthritis sufferers are malnourished.[72] By restoring optimal nutritional levels to the diet, these arthritis sufferers can benefit to a greater extent than they would otherwise.

A potent vitamin, mineral and phytochemical formula, together with antioxidants, enzymes, and herbs such as ginger and turmeric, is extremely helpful. This type of broad-based support can help to account for many deficiencies. "I recommend a simple multivitamin to correct nutrient deficiencies," says Ranjit Chandra, M.D., twice nominated for the Nobel Prize in medicine, holder of five honorary doctorates and a visiting professor at universities on four continents.[73] "In our studies in Newfoundland, 35 to 40 percent of older people have deficiencies." What's more, adds Dr. Chandra, "it isn't just one nutrient that is deficient." Yet, he adds, "finding out which ones are deficient is impractical and very expensive because you'd have to measure both dietary intake and blood levels of 20 different nutrients." Using a broad-based formula daily is the practical approach. It covers your bases to insure you won't be deficient in a wide range of nutrients. Several excellent brands are available.

Always work with your health professional, especially if you are on any type of medication.

### Testing for Dietary Deficiencies

Should you be tested for nutrient levels in your blood or other tissues? Testing can be helpful—and tricky. A high level of magnesium in the blood, for instance, may not be a good sign because it may indicate that the mineral is *not* being taken up by cells themselves.

It is extremely important to do a complete spectrum of testing for levels of vitamins, minerals, amino acids and other nutrients in the blood. Very often, health care professionals do some tests—but not all. A key link in solving nutritional deficiencies could be missing.

A 61-year-old San Francisco woman, who had been very active socially, playing tennis and entertaining almost every day, came to her doctor complaining of stiffened, swollen ankles. Her other doctor had done some scattershot testing.

The symptoms seemed to be precisely like those of osteoarthritis, but they had emerged quite suddenly. Could there be another cause?

Her new doctor ordered a vitamin blood test that the other doctor had skipped. It revealed she was low in pantothenic acid (vitamin B-5), and that made all the difference in the world. As she put more pantothenic acid into her supplement program, her ankles returned to normal and she was able to resume her active tennis life.

## Take a Daily Multiple Formula

We strongly recommend a daily broad-based vitamin and mineral formula for extra nutritional insurance (see chart) which should supply a wide range of antioxidants (many of which are discussed later in this chapter). In addition, we also recommend a separate antioxidant supplement to help curb the damage caused by the release of excessive amounts of free radicals due to inflammation of the joints. The amounts we've listed are rough estimates of what a supplement should provide daily as nutritional insurance. It is in addition to, not instead of a whole foods diet. Some nutrients, such as black cohosh extract for women and saw palmetto berry extract for men, may also be supplemented in larger amounts as single, high-potency, pharmaceutically standardized nutrients for specific maladies such as menopausal symptoms or benign prostatic hyperplasia (enlarged prostate). Be sure all vitamins are, insofar as possible, naturally sourced.

## Recommended General Amounts
## for Daily Supplement Program

| Nutrient | Daily Recommended Amount |
| --- | --- |
| **Vitamins** | |
| Vitamin A (beta-carotene) | 15,000 IU |
| Vitamin A (retinol) | 2,500 IU |
| Mixed carotenes (including lycopene) | 5 mg |
| Vitamin E (d-alpha tocopherol succinate) | 200 IU |
| Vitamin D | 100 IU |
| Vitamin C | 300 mg |
| Vitamin B-1 (thiamine) | 60 mg |
| Vitamin B-2 (riboflavin) | 60 mg |
| Vitamin B-3 (niacin/niacinamide) | 90 mg |
| Vitamin B-6 (pyridoxine) | 90 mg |

| Nutrient | Daily Recommended Amount |
|---|---|
| Pantothenic acid (d-calcium pantothenate) | 30 mg |
| Folic acid | 800 mcg |
| Vitamin B-12 (cyanocobalamin or methylcobalamin) | 800 mcg |
| Biotin | 600 mcg |
| Inositol | 30 mg |
| Choline | 30 mg |
| Para-aminobenzoic acid (PABA) | 30 mg |
| Vitamin K | 60 mcg |

**Minerals**

| | |
|---|---|
| Calcium citrate | 200–400 mg |
| Magnesium (aspartate, chloride) | 300–400 mg |
| Potassium (aspartate) | 99 mg |
| Zinc (picolinate) | 20 mg |
| Manganese | 5 mg |
| Copper | 1 mg |
| Chromium (polynicotine) | 200 mcg |
| Selenium (selenomethionine) | 200 mcg |
| Molybdenum | 25 mcg |
| Vanadium sulfate | 50 mcg |
| Boron | 3 mg |
| Silica | 1 mg |

**Herbs**

| | |
|---|---|
| Iodine (kelp) | 300 mcg |

| *Nutrient* | *Daily Recommended Amount* |
|---|---|
| Ginger root | 30 mg |
| Green tea | 30 mg |
| | |
| **For Women** | |
| Dong quai extract | 30 mg |
| Licorice root extract | 30 mg |
| Chaste tree berry extract | 15 mg |
| Fennel seed extract | 15 mg |
| | |
| **For Men** | |
| Muira puama extract | 30 mg |
| Saw palmetto berry extract | 30 mg |
| Korean ginseng extract | 15 mg |

# Take a Daily Antioxidant Formula

We also recommend a daily antioxidant formula for added defenses against inflammation. A mass of evidence proves that the chemicals in fruits and vegetables truly allow people to live longer, healthier lives. The powerful molecules locked in fruits, vegetables and other nutrient-rich plant foods and herbs are called phytochemicals (from the Greek *phyto* for plants). Phytochemicals have been proven to help maintain healthy cholesterol levels, blood pressure, joint mobility, vision, memory and prostate function. Yet nine of ten people simply don't eat enough fresh fruits and vegetables to get all of the powerful benefits from phytochemicals that they should. Phytochemicals are neither vitamins nor minerals but are equally, if not more powerful, in the health benefits that they offer.

To be sure, supplements cannot take the place of a good diet, but they can help to make up for a poor diet. What's more, antioxidants, whose job is to scavenge harmful free radicals, work better together than separately. So it's important to supplement a wide variety of antioxidant nutrients. Researchers in the Department of Food Science and Technology at the University of California, Davis, found that experimental animals receiving the greatest variety of antioxidants do best in fighting premature aging.[74] Single antioxidants also work, but a diverse variety works even better. When it comes to nutritional superheroes like antioxidants, variety is not only the spice—but also the extender—of life.

Those antioxidants studied at the University of California included vitamins, minerals and phytochemicals such as beta-carotene, vitamin C, vitamin E, selenium, coenzyme Q10, acetylcysteine and catechins found in green tea. Fortunately, these powerful protectors are now available in nutritional supplements that can be used daily.

Even the prestigious *Journal of the National Cancer Institute* includes research into phytochemicals in almost every issue. Consumers who wish to be on the cutting edge of safe and beneficial trends in health should act on this information now. Research into phytochemicals is awakening a slumbering giant about to be unleashed for the good of your health. There are many excellent antioxidant formulas on the market.

A good antioxidant/phytochemical formula should look like this:

| Nutrient | Daily Recommended Amount | |
|---|---|---|
| **Vitamins** | | |
| Vitamin A (beta-carotene) | 10,000 | IU |
| Vitamin E (D-alpha tocopherol) | 200 | IU |
| Vitamin C | 500 | mg |
| Zinc (picolinate) | 15 | mg |
| Manganese | 15 | mg |
| Vitamin B-2 (riboflavin) | 6 | mg |
| Selenium (L-selenomethionine) | 200 | mcg |
| N-acetylcysteine | 100 | mg |
| Cabbage extract | 100 | mg |
| Garlic extract | 100 | mg |
| Ginger root extract | 100 | mg |
| Green tea extract | 100 | mg |
| Curcuma root extract (turmeric) | 50 | mg |
| Grapeseed extract | 10 | mg |

Now that we've taken care of the basics, let's discuss nutrients that have shown special benefits for people with arthritis.

# Fish Oils

We discussed the value of fish oils, as derived from a whole food diet, in Chapter 7. The evidence that fish oils can benefit rheumatoid arthritis sufferers is so strong that we would like to see *all* of our rheumatoid arthritis (RA) patients eating more seafood and/or taking fish oil capsules. We performed extensive Medline data searches and found that many clinical studies offer strong proof of their efficacy.

Investigations from Europe, the United States and Australia have described consistent improvement in tender joint scores with many investigators also observing improvements in morning stiffness. Recent studies also suggest that some patients are able to discontinue NSAIDs while taking fish oils.

One recent study done to determine whether dietary supplementation with fish oil could replace NSAIDs in patients with rheumatoid arthritis also looked at the clinical efficacy of high-dose dietary omega-3 fatty acid fish oil supplementation in RA patients and the effect of fish oil supplements on the production of inflammation-related cytokines in this population.[75] Sixty-six patients entered a double-blind, placebo-controlled, prospective study of fish oil supplementation while taking diclofenac (75 mg twice a day).

Patients took either 130 mg/kg/day of omega-3 fatty acids or 9 capsules/day of corn oil. Serum levels of the proinflammatory cytokines, including interleukin-1 beta (IL-1 beta), IL-2, IL-6 and IL-8 and tumor necrosis factor alpha, were measured. In the group taking fish oil, there were significant decreases from baseline in the mean number of tender joints, duration of morning stiffness, physician's and patient's evaluation of arthritis activity and the physician's evaluation of pain. In patients taking corn oil, no clinical parameters improved from baseline. The decrease in the number of tender joints remained significant eight weeks after discontinuing treatment. Some patients who took fish oil were able to discontinue NSAIDs without experiencing a disease flare up. Levels of inflammatory cytokines also decreased significantly. Indeed, there was a direct correlation between the lowest levels of proinflammatory cytokines and the patients whose condition improved the most.

In a 1993 study from the *British Journal of Rheumatology*, patients were instructed to slowly reduce their NSAID dosage providing there was no worsening of their symptoms. There was a significant reduction in NSAID usage in patients taking the fish oil when compared with placebo from month three.[76]

Michael Murray, N.D., observes, "Over a dozen follow-up studies consistently demonstrate positive benefits. In addition to improving symptoms (morning stiffness and joint tenderness), fish oil supplementation produces favorable changes in suppressing the production of inflammatory compounds secreted by white blood cells."[77]

The optimal daily dosage is 10 one-gram capsules, each supplying 180 mg of EPA or 1.8 *grams* of EPA daily.[78]

Women who are pregnant and others who wish to minimize their exposure to environmental pollutants may consider supplementing their diet with flaxseed oil, as fish oil capsules may have small amounts of contamination from pesticides and industrial chemicals.[79] However, before you start to panic about small amounts of contamination, it is important to maintain perspective. The benefits conferred by fish oil supplements to arthritis sufferers and also to persons suffering other forms of inflammatory disease, as well as for protection against heart disease and circulatory problems, clearly outweigh any small risks these contaminants may pose. Still, the nutritional industry should take all means necessary to reduce contamination in fish oil supplements.

# B Complex Vitamins

Pantothenic acid (vitamin B-5), a member of the B complex family of vitamins, has been found in particular to be deficient in arthritis sufferers. The level of deficiency is directly related to the severity of symptoms.[80] Moreover, this nutrient seems to work for both rheumatoid arthritis and osteoarthritis.[81, 82] One study found that *as much as two grams* daily of pantothenic acid resulted in significant reduction in the duration of morning stiffness, degree of disability and severity of pain.[82] The elderly, in particular, may be deficient in this important nutrient.

Vitamin B-12 is the vitamin most often deficient in pain disorders. Frequently the blood level in patients with chronic pain or nervous system problems is 200 to 400 pg/ml. The normal frame in the United States has been listed as 300–2,500 pg/ml, but the Pacific Rim lists their low end of normal at 600 pg/ml. It's clear that many American patients with clinical pain syndromes have levels well into the abnormal range if compared to the Asian standard.

Vitamin B-6 has also been studied quite extensively in regard to compressive syndromes such as carpal tunnel. The results from these studies have been quite prominent in showing that pyridoxine is essential for normal nerve health, and hence its efficacy in various pain states has been crucial.

## Vitamin C

Many reasons can be found to supplement with extra vitamin C. For one, vitamin C helps to reduce inflammation and histamine levels, as well as enhance the body's antioxidant activity. Vitamin C's antioxidant properties are vital to tissue repair and building immunity. The adage that more is better has been documented quite extensively, with Linus Pauling taking nearly 20 grams a day and living to his mid-90s with full vitality. Vitamin C is essential to building healthy connective tissues.[83] Rheumatoid arthritis patients may especially suffer from low vitamin C levels.[84] As so many arthritis patients are adults, it is important to note that as one ages, the body's vitamin C levels are commonly low, resulting in altered collagen synthesis and compromised connective tissue repair.[83] We recommend a high intake of vitamin C-rich foods plus supplements of 500–3,000 mg daily. A high intake of vitamin C can help reduce pain and swelling and also nourish connective tissues in the joints.[84, 85] Interestingly, vitamin C, together with bioflavonoids, enhances the anti-inflammatory effects of enzymes like bromelain.[86] In fact, this combination of vitamin C—augmented by flavonoids such as those in grapeseed extract together with bromelain— demonstrates "a more complete spectrum of action" against inflammation than typically prescribed medical drugs.[86]

## Vitamin E

Vitamin E may help arthritis sufferers because it is a prostaglandin inhibitor (much like NSAIDs such as aspirin).[87] Other researchers, however, believe its beneficial effect is due to its free radical scavenging capabilities and its stabilizing influence on cell membranes. Others attribute vitamin E's benefits to its inhibition of enzymes that destroy cartilage and its stimulating effect on cartilage cell production.[88]

Two studies indicate vitamin E combined with selenium can help to improve health in rheumatoid arthritis patients.[89, 90] The best dosage of vitamin E is from 400–1,200 IU daily, with most studies showing benefits at around 600 to 800 IUs. Vitamin E is especially important to supplement, as its availability in the modern food supply is limited to a few concentrated high-fat sources such as wheat germ and soybean oils. Wheat germ cereal is an excellent source, but still could never provide the amount found to be optimal in major clinical trials.

# Minerals

Among minerals most consistently shown to be helpful in chronic pain states are magnesium, selenium, zinc, and copper.

## Magnesium

Magnesium may be particularly helpful for fibromyalgia. Supplementing with 300 to 600 mg of magnesium malate daily has shown very good benefits.[91]

## Selenium

One of the key roles that selenium plays in supporting underlying health in cases of arthritis is by acting as a mineral building block for the free radical scavenging enzyme glutathione peroxidase, which is found at low levels in many arthritis patients.[92]

Our recommended dosage is 200 mcg daily of a highly bioavailable form of selenium called selenomethionine.

## Zinc

One of zinc's important roles in the body is to stimulate conversion of alpha-linoleic acid (found in flaxseed oil) to gamma-linoleic acid and eventually to EPA, which is very good for the body's inflammatory processes and joint health, particularly in cases of rheumatoid arthritis. Very often rheumatoid arthritis patients suffer zinc deficiencies. Murray and Pizzorno report that several studies show slight benefits to rheumatoid arthritis sufferers who supplement their diets with zinc.[92] Zinc is also essential to the body for making collagen.[93] We recommend 20 to 45 mg daily.

## *Copper*

The use of copper bracelets for arthritis may be valid. Some forms of copper, especially copper aspirinate (salicylate), have been shown to work better as an anti-inflammatory and pain reliever than pure aspirin. Copper bracelets work by providing copper which is absorbed through the skin and converted into a usable form in the body. Copper aids the body in producing a major free radical scavenger, superoxide dismutase. Those who take a standard multiple vitamin and mineral formula will get a sufficient amount of copper (3 mg).

# Amino Acids

Amino acids are the building blocks of proteins, which play many different roles in the body. Although the body manufactures many amino acids, eight are considered to be available only via diet; these are the essential amino acids. Amino acids are generally overlooked in cases of arthritis; two, however, are important to know about because their benefits have been well documented.

## *D, L-phenylalanine (DLPA)*

This form of the amino acid phenylalanine, which combines the natural D form with the synthetic and mirror-opposite L form, is able to penetrate the blood-brain barrier and inhibit the body's destruction of painkilling endorphins. DLPA has been shown to produce extremely excellent pain-relieving results in several clinical trials conducted by members of the Department of Pharmacology and Anesthesiology at the University of Chicago Medical School. The usual dosage is 400 mg three times daily. The effect is cumulative but, for many patients, it is quite pronounced and has provided help when NSAIDs have failed.

### S-adenosyl-methionine (SAM)

Another promising amino acid-based nutrient, SAM is a sulfur-rich nutrient that seems to provide excellent pain relief. A 1985 double-blind clinical trial found SAM was able to work better than ibuprofen for hip-related osteoarthritis.[94] Other studies confirm its pain-relieving abilities in fibromyalgia as well.[95]

Using SAM requires special strategies as it can cause nausea and gastrointestinal disturbances.[95] Murray advises starting at a dosage of 200 mg twice daily on the first day, increasing to 400 mg twice daily on day three and 400 mg three times daily by day ten, staying with the full dosage of 1,200 mg daily until symptoms are reduced, then gradually lowering the dosage and tapering to a maintenance dosage of 200 mg twice daily.[95] The dosage for fibromyalgia is 200–400 mg two to three times daily.[95]

## Oral Combination Enzymes

Also known as oral systemic combination enzymes, these powerful substances can have a profound effect on immune-mediated diseases. It isn't surprising, therefore, that they've been demonstrated to be extremely beneficial in cases of rheumatoid arthritis. Excellent results using the patented enzyme formula Wobenzym N were noted by researchers in a 1985 report in *Zeitschr. f. Rheumatologie*. In this study, patients took eight Wobenzym N tablets four times daily. Sixty-two percent of patients improved.[96] A 1988 report in *Natur und Ganzheits-medizin* showed that the same formula can prevent further flare-ups and helps to lower levels of inflammatory-related circulating immune complexes in rheumatoid arthritis patients.[97] A study published in the same journal in 1988 noted that Wobenzym has demonstrated similar benefits to gold therapy, but without toxic side effects.[98] Patients may be required to take up to 30 Wobenzym tablets daily, but the results and the product's excellent safety profile make their use extremely worthwhile among people with rheumatoid arthritis.

Combination oral enzymes help in other autoimmune diseases. Thus, they are particularly helpful to persons with SLE. Enzymes help to dissolve circulating immune complexes and antibodies that cause severe inflammation in cases of SLE. According to D.A. Lopez, M.D., associate clinical professor of medicine at the University of California at San Diego Medical School and co-author of *Enzymes: The Fountain of Life*, animals suffering from this inflammatory condition, when given combination enzymes, have shown significant improvement. Enzymes may be particularly important for SLE sufferers for another reason: they've been strongly shown to help prevent kidney disease and failure, both of which are commonly associated with SLE, according to August Heidland, M.D., and coinvestigators report-ing in a 1997 issue of *Kidney International*.[99]

The enzyme mixture most thoroughly documented to help retard or prevent kidney failure among SLE patients, and the one used in virtually every study to which the *Kidney International* report refers, is Wobenzym N and its closely related derivatives, all produced by Mucos Pharma GmbH & Co., of Germany. The third leading over-the-counter preparation in Germany, Wobenzym N is now available in health food stores in the United States. It may be particularly important for both rheumatoid arthritis and SLE patients (see Resources for information on where to obtain Wobenzym N).

## Cetyl Myristoleate

Cetyl myristoleate is a potentially beneficial, newly recognized substance for the treatment of inflammatory-related arthritis. Cetyl myristoleate, which may be both animal or plant derived, first came to prominence when an experimental study was published by Harry W. Diehl in the March 1994 *Journal of Pharmaceutical Sciences* that showed it totally protected against artificially induced inflammatory arthritis. Diehl, who worked 40 years at the National Institutes of Health Laboratory of Chemistry of the National Institute of Arthritis, Metabolic and Digestive Diseases, began his research in 1962, spurred on by his observation that mice appeared to be virtually immune from naturally occurring arthritis. By 1964, he determined that a substance in mice protected them against naturally occurring arthritis. This immunity factor was eventually isolated and determined to be cetyl myristoleate, which is also commonly found in beavers and sperm whales.

Cetyl myristoleate was studied against placebo and also combined with glucosamine hydrochloride, sea cucumber and hydrolyzed cartilage against placebo in an unpublished clinical trial conducted by Humberto Siemandi at Hospital SM, Rosarito Beach, Baja California, Mexico, under the auspices of the Joint European Hospital Studies Program. The dosage was 18 grams of cetyl myristoleate given orally.

In all parameters, including doctor- and patient-reported evaluations of pain and mobility, as well as other clinical and laboratory analyses, patients receiving cetyl myristoleate did better than placebo. Patients receiving cetyl myristoleate with the additional substances, glucosamine hydrochloride, sea cucumber and hydrolyzed cartilage, however, did even better. We believe that more clinical research on cetyl myristoleate will be required before it can be recommended in the treatment of inflammatory-related arthritis.

## Prolotherapy

The word *prolotherapy* is short for proliferation therapy, because prolotherapy causes the proliferation, growth and formation of new ligament and tendon tissues in areas where these have become weakened due to injury. Ligaments are the structural "rubber bands" that hold bones to bones in the joints, while tendons join muscles to bones. Unfortunately, both may become torn or otherwise injured.

Prolotherapy is used for many different types of musculoskeletal pain, including arthritis, back pain, neck pain, fibromyalgia, sports injuries, unresolved whiplash injuries, carpal tunnel syndrome, torn tendons, ligaments and cartilage, and degenerated or herniated discs.

The concept behind prolotherapy is that a small, mild stimulus, such as the injection of reconstructive nutrients, causes dilation of blood vessels and a migration of healing cells to the injured areas. These healing cells help to lay down collagen, the structural protein of the joint matrix.

In this therapy, a slender needle is inserted into the area where the tendon or ligament attaches to the bone. Various substances can be used separately or combined, such as calcium gluconate, dextrose, zinc or an extract from cod liver fish oil, also known as sodium morrhuate, in a base of saline with a local anesthetic.

Each treatment results in more and more tissue being laid down in damaged areas; with each treatment, joints continue to become stronger. Snapping, clicking and popping sounds decrease, patients enjoy greater endurance and can once again participate in more activities. Results from successful clinical studies have been reported in several prestigious journals and books, including one by M.J. Ongley and coinvestigators in the July 18, 1987 *Lancet*. Prolotherapy is best performed by an experienced health professional. Its benefits can be enhanced with the use of patented glucosamine sulfate, according to our own clinical experience with patients. (See Resources for a web site dedicated to prolotherapy.)

# Phytochemical/Herbal Remedies

There are multiple herbs with individual constituent chemicals that have been found helpful for the restoration of optimal well-being in patients with chronic pain syndromes such as arthritis.

### *Turmeric*

Also known as *Curcuma longa*, turmeric is a potent anti-inflammatory. Jean Carper reports in *Food—Your Miracle Medicine* that its active ingredient, curcumin, "is an anti-inflammatory agent on a par with cortisone and has reduced inflammation in animals and symptoms of rheumatoid arthritis in humans."[100] It has been noted that 1,200 mg of the active ingredient in turmeric, curcumin, is the equivalent of 300 mg of phenylbutazone.[101]

## Bromelain

An enzyme derived from the pineapple plant, bromelain is a potent anti-inflammatory agent on a par with aspirin (but much safer) and one whose benefits have been suggested in numerous clinical studies.[102] Bromelain was shown to reduce joint swelling in cases of arthritis and has worked where long-term steroids have not. Moreover, bromelain is absorbable from the gastrointestinal tract if placed in enterically coated capsules.[103] Unlike medical drugs used for inflammation associated with arthritis, the health-promoting effects of bromelain are without dangerous complications.

## Willow Bark

Willow bark is another natural source of substances that inhibit inflammation-causing prostaglandins. Willow bark is a rich source of salicylate, the world's oldest, most revered nutrient for maintaining healthy, inflammation-free joints.[104]

## Licorice Root

A complement to bromelain and willow bark, licorice root's active ingredient, glycyrrhizin, has also demonstrated potent anti-inflammatory powers. In fact, licorice root concentrate effectively inhibits some of the most potent inflammatory agents in the body.[105]

## Pycnogenol

The paramount players here are antioxidants called proantho-cyanidins or pycnogenols. Frequently called pine bark or grape-seed extract, pycnogenols have been helpful with various arthritis disorders. These substances help to relieve inflammation by rebalancing the body's production of histamines, which act as proinflammatory agents in the body. They also help to protect the body's connective tissue.[106]

## Feverfew

Known as *Tanacetum parthenium,* feverfew is an excellent herbal anti-inflammatory which has long been used in traditional healing for relieving fever, migraine and arthritis. Several studies have validated its headache relieving and prophylactic effects. Feverfew inhibits pro-inflammatory compounds.

## Ginger, Cloves and Garlic

Consuming liberal amounts of ginger, cloves and garlic in your foods may also help to relieve some of the inflammation associated with rheumatoid arthritis. These spices help to block inflammatory-related prostaglandins and leukotrienes. Be sure to add these spices to your meals at the end of cooking and cook them at as low a temperature as possible; high cooking tempera-tures may destroy some of their most important constituents.

### China Root and Wild Yam Root

China root and wild yam root are two ancient, yet newly discovered, herbal arthritis remedies that have been traditionally used for centuries among the indigenous peoples of Central America, reports Dr. Rosita Arvigo, D.N, president and a cofounder of the Ix Chel Tropical Research Foundation in Cayo, Belize, and Michael J. Balick, Ph.D., director and curator of economic botany at the Institute of Economic Botany of The New York Botanical Gardens.[107] China root is a thorny vine that grows up into the forest canopy with an underground red tuber. For use, the natives chop and boil a small handful of China root in three cups of water. To use wild yam root, natives make a hot tea from the tuber and drink three times daily before meals. (See Resources for sources of these rainforest remedies.)

# What about Chondroitin Sulfate?

Made up of chains of sugars, chondroitin sulfates are found in cartilage, where they create tiny reservoirs to attract and hold water in the proteoglycan mortar. They help to bring water, shape and cushioning to cartilage.

Chondroitin sulfates inhibit destructive enzymes that break down cartilage and prevent the carrying of nutrients into the cartilage; they stimulate synthesis of proteoglycans, glycosaminoglycans and collagen, which make up healthy cartilage. They are manufactured from healthy cartilage.

Chondroitin sulfates recently received a great deal of attention in *The Arthritis Cure* by Jason Theodosakis, et al. We take issue with the claims presented in this book.

Chondroitin sulfate is an extremely large molecule and has been conclusively proven *not* to be well absorbed in the body when taken orally. In the journal *Rheumatology International*, A. Baici, of the Department of Rheumatology, University Hospital, Zurich, Switzerland, and coinvestigators reported that chondroitin sulfate has never been shown to be absorbed intact.[108]

> Considering all of the experimental evidence discussed above, it can be concluded that chondroitin sulfate is not absorbed as an intact molecule from the mammalian digestive tract and that the bulk of this glycosaminoglycan, when administered orally, is eliminated in the feces, either intact or after partial degradation. Therefore, any possible beneficial effect deriving from the oral administration of chondroitin sulfate to human beings must be sought outside the biological actions attributed to the intact molecule being absorbed through the digestive tract. The hypothesis of an accumulation of chondroitin sulfate in articular cartilage after oral administration has never been demonstrated and makes little sense from a biological point of view.[108]

*The Arthritis Cure* purports that chondroitin sulfate must be used with glucosamine sulfate for the full effect. This statement is without clinical merit.

The majority of the studies actually cited in *The Arthritis Cure* have nothing to do with oral chondroitin sulfate. In fact, one from 1974 used injectable chondroitin with 28 patients who were suffering severe osteoarthritis.[109] The results were not relevant to the consumer who consumes chondroitin sulfate *orally*. A 1987 Argentine study looked at chondroitin sulfates compared to a placebo and, while there was an improvement, the form used was injectable.[110] A study published in 1991 from the University of

Genoa and also cited in *The Arthritis Cure*, notes that researchers compared the effects of injections of chondroitin, together with injections of a nonsteroidal anti-inflammatory drug, to a placebo in a double-blind study.[111] There was a gradual diminishing of pain, and gradually the chondroitin users were able to receive fewer drugs. Again, this was an injectable form of chondroitin sulfate and not relevant to the consumer. Another 1991 study, from the University of Naples, involved 200 patients ranging in age from their 50s to their 70s.[112] The results were positive, but this study used both injectable and oral chondroitin, leaving a question as to whether there was a cross-over effect from the combination. A 1992 study focusing on oral chondroitin sulfates found improvement, but the patients were given other pain-killing drugs along with it, obscuring the true effect and again leaving in doubt whether there was a synergistic effect.[113]

That leaves two studies looking at oral chondroitin sulfate alone. In 1986, a French study using oral chondroitin sulfates found that it helped heal arthritic cartilage better than pain medication.[114] A 1996 study from the *Journal of Rheumatology* assessed the clinical efficacy of chondroitin sulfate in comparison with diclofenac. Patients treated with the NSAID showed prompt and plain reduction of clinical symptoms, which, however, reappeared after the end of treatment; in the chondroitin group, the therapeutic response appeared later in time but lasted for up to three months after the end of treatment.[115]

Of seven major studies on chondroitin sulfate, only two used the oral form alone.

What's more, no studies were cited that actually examined the combination of glucosamine sulfate and chondroitin sulfate. We conducted an extensive Medline computer data base search on results of studies using a combination of chondroitin and glucosamine sulfates. Not a single study has ever been published that we were able to locate. In his foreword to *The Arthritis Cure*,

Amal Das, M.D., admits that he is "currently conducting the first human double-blind, prospective, randomized study of these substances in the United States . . . with a total of 100 people."[116]

Chondroitin sulfate, says medical author Ray Sahelian, M.D. understatedly, has "very limited research."[117] A recent report in *U.S. News & World Report* notes the peculiar absence of hard data in *The Arthritis Cure*. Speaking of the studies cited in the book, the news magazine observed: "None of them tested chondroitin sulfate and glucosamine together."[118]

Based on anecdotes alone and without a single study to back the combination, the nutritional industry jumped on the chondroitin sulfate bandwagon. There is no credible evidence to support use of this combination.

## Bottom Line

- Take a daily quality multiple vitamin, mineral and phytochemical supplement that supplies extra amounts of herbal antioxidants such as green tea and turmeric.
- Fish oils and enzymes are important supplements for rheumatoid arthritis and should be used with the patented form of glucosamine sulfate.
- Other agents, such as specific vitamins, minerals and herbs may also help.
- Be sure to work with your health care professional when taking nutritional supplements.

# 10

## Becoming Who You Were Always Meant to Be

Uncontrolled arthritis pain is a national tragedy. We can do better. We need to find out what causes arthritis and what aggravates it. We need to pinpoint specific therapies that will either reverse or retard its progression, lessen pain and improve functionality.

Unfortunately, however, there are hurdles. It is unlikely that your physician will sit down with you and talk about options, particularly as they relate to nutritional supplementation or lifestyle changes. It is important to find a physician that will take the time, often an hour or more, and thoroughly review what you can do to begin healing. The case histories we've shared occurred between real physicians and real patients who were in *pain*, but these were doctors who focused on patients, not insurance forms.

In America today a small, powerful medical movement, perhaps not as large as we would like, is pushing back from polypharmacy and focusing more on prevention, wellness and natural healing pathways. A resource section has been appended so you can find a medical practitioner with this philosophy.

The road to wellness is not easy in a country like America where there is so little support for those who are suffering. It is also not cheap. While glucosamine sulfate costs less than most arthritis drugs on a monthly basis, individuals on a limited income without insurance coverage, will feel the economic pinch. Programs designed to reduce stress and enhance flexibility, endurance and strength usually involve highly trained individuals who work either one-on-one or with small groups. Their services are usually less expensive than a formal physical therapy program, but again, if there is no coverage, these programs can be costly.

One must also form a new frame of mind regarding wellness. This means surmounting the denial, anger and depression that usually accompanies the chronic pain of arthritis. Healing requires an attitudinal shift, a shift toward gratefulness for being alive, for the enjoyment of friends and family, an acceptance that life is a gift and that we were not made to be immortal. We have personally seen some arthritis patients transcend their pain, reaching out to others and giving instead of receiving. Their pain, in a sense, is a gain, in that these patients focus more on the transcendant than on the urgent; they make pain a prism instead of a prison.

"As far as I'm concerned, wholeness and spirituality are synonymous," notes author John Bradshaw. He might have added that wholeness, spirituality and health are synonymous. Yet in an industrialized world, where technology has become the dominant force in medicine and where mind and spirit are divorced from the holiness of our bodies, it is no wonder that so many people are unhappy, unhealthy and spiritually depleted. This loss of connectedness to a greater reality, is as sickening to the human body as a fatty diet, environmental pollution, tobacco and other well-publicized causes of disease. Yet we pay little attention to this aspect of sickness.

In society, people are not freer by day to communicate their innermost feelings, hurts, sorrows, fears or joy. At night, people are so addicted to television and noncommunication that there is no way they can purge themselves of the day's build-up of emotional stress and physical tension. Talking is replaced by canned laughter. This bottling-up effect has led to massive stress and a sense of hopelessness and apathy. These, in turn, have created even greater health problems, including cancer, heart disease and arthritis.

Famed neuropsychologist Kenneth R. Pelletier of the University of California School of Medicine, notes that stress-related psychological and physiological disorders have become the number-one social and health problem in America over the last decade. He goes on to point out that stress-induced disorders have long since replaced epidemics of infectious disease as the major medical problem of the modern era.[119]

## The Arthritic Personality

R.H. Moos studied over 5,000 rheumatoid arthritis sufferers and isolated several personality traits, for example, which differentiated them from arthritis-free persons, including their tendency to be "self-sacrificing, masochistic, conforming, self-conscious, shy, inhibited, perfectionistic, and interested in sports."[120]

Arthritic patients typically were nervous, tense, worried, moody, depressed and typically had mothers who had rejected them and fathers who were unduly strict. They had difficulty expressing anger. Anger, anxiety, depression, compliance-subservience, conservatism, security-seeking, shyness and introversion were also found to be more prevalent among such sufferers. Sufferers who were more anxious and depressed, isolated, alienated and introverted were also more likely to suffer a worse prognosis.

In 1969, George Solomon observed that many people have the

rheumatoid arthritis factor but that it was their psychological health that either created their vulnerability to this factor or did not.[121]

## Herbs for Pain, Sleep, and Mood

Because pain hurts, interferes with sleep and provokes anxiety, a variety of natural substances have emerged to restore sleep or peace of mind. These include valerian root, passionflower, hops and chamomile which are mild sedatives. The pineal hormone melatonin can also enhance sleep.

*Hypericum perforatum* (St. John's wort) has well-known antidepressant and analgesic properties regarding neuropathic pain and, particularly, slice injuries to the fingers. In its more traditional herbal role, it balances and harmonizes mood, hence acting as a natural antidepressant. Try this herb before using medically prescribed mood altering or antidepressant drugs.

A 1996 report in the *British Medical Journal* is only the latest to extol this powerful herb's antidepressant activities. "Fortunately, more doctors are starting to recommend it for depression," says health author Ray Sahelian, M.D. "In those who are young, generally 50 years old or less, and who don't suffer from suicidal tendencies or severe depression, St. John's wort should be the first medicine to be tried."[122]

Seek a standardized dosage of St. John's wort that provides 300 mg per capsule and is certified to contain 0.3% hypericin (900 mcg per capsule). Take one capsule three times a day with meals. If sleep is disrupted, take two capsules in the morning and one at midday. Adjust the dosage to your individual needs; side effects are mild and transient, and may include dizziness, nausea, tiredness and dry mouth in a small percentage of people.

# Tools for Healing

## *Keep a Journal*

Keeping a journal or diary will bolster your commitment to a healthy diet and exercise program. Journals are an important method of self-exploration and personal growth.

In your health journal, you might want to start by writing about your feelings about your arthritis or other health conditions. Be honest. Be descriptive and detailed. Also keep a daily food and exercise diary and record how your body is improving as you dedicate yourself to your physical and spiritual well-being.

Some may prefer to use a computer for journal keeping, but be sure to keep the printed pages in a notebook so that you can leaf through them easily in a relaxed atmosphere away from your computer monitor. Others may choose to put pen to paper and keep a journal in a specially designated notebook. Either way is fine. Use your journal as a method of self-exploration for *all* of your life, well beyond your concerns about arthritis. Use it to write down how you see yourself at your best and to map out all the goals of your new life—the life that you're starting today because you want to be better and healthier than ever.

# Stress Triggers

You will also feel better as you begin to deal more effectively with other stressful influences in your life. Stress is often a very real symbol of our loss of connectedness with our spiritual quest. Our lives are out of balance, or, perhaps we are not living our lives in accordance with out deepest needs and values. To deal effectively with stress, you may want to use your journal to conduct a personal self-appraisal of your own stress triggers. It is also important to recognize that stress triggers are often overlapping, fueling each other. Financial difficulties can create relationship difficulties. Illness can become financially devastating and test any relationship. Experts have found that five areas of people's lives seem to produce the greatest stress. Most people will enjoy better health by addressing these problem areas in their lives as soon as possible.

## Physical

Air, noise and light pollution can create extreme stress, turning homes and workplaces into pressure chambers. Overcrowding in urban living situations also creates stress.

## Job-related

Deadline pressures on the job, the constant sense of competition, an individual's poor relationship with a difficult boss and working at a job that is neither meaningful nor enjoyable are all major stresses.

When we lose a job, major stresses occur. University of Michigan researcher Sidney Cobb studied 100 auto-paint factory workers starting from six weeks before their jobs were to be terminated, following them for two years. Incidence of hypertension, peptic ulcers, arthritis and psychosomatic disorders all increased. Moreover, three wives were hospitalized with rare peptic ulcers.

## Financial

Money difficulties are a number-one cause of divorce, domestic violence and worry.

## Relationship

A difficult time with a lover, mate, child or friend can create unyielding stress. A death in the family or loss of a relationship can also be stressful.

## Social change

Marriage, pregnancy, job changes or moving can also become excessively stressful if focused in too short a period of time. Researchers have found that illnesses tend to occur at times when clusters of such major events have occurred in people's lives within a fairly short time frame.

You can overcome stress by making decisions and sticking with them. That may require changing jobs or moving to a less urbanized area of the country where there is less crowding and the cost of living is less expensive.

The point is to make the decision right now to start examining your deepest needs and to make sure you take small steps daily to fulfill these needs. Although not all stress is harmful, remember that when stress turns to *distress*, it is time to take action.

Losing mobility and irritated by constant pain, some people may lose hope and faith, but, the healing powers within your body are there. You just need to nourish them with the proper nutrients, dietary and lifestyle changes.

Be patient, but don't give up. With proper dietary changes, emphasizing more fresh fruits and vegetables and whole grains, adequate pure water, proper exercise, glucosamine sulfate and other supplements as needed, you can do something about your arthritis. That is the positive message. There is hope. There is no need to suffer. You can reverse this condition and improve. That is our ironclad promise.

You chose to come through the door with us. Now choose to go back through the door this time as the person you were always meant to be—with your health restored.

# Glossary

**Active movements.** Movements specifically initiated by the patient.

**Amino acids.** Any of a class of organic compounds containing at least one amino group (derived from ammonia) and used as a building block for protein in the human body.

**Analgesic.** Pain relief medication, usually without cartilage-regenerating properties.

**Antibody.** Protein molecule produced by the immune system's B-cells as a primary immune defense. These combine with antigens.

**Antigen.** Substance that stimulates the body's production of antibodies.

**Antioxidant.** Substance that scavenges free radicals and reduces oxidation of body tissues and cells.

**Arachidonic acid.** A type of prostaglandin found almost entirely in animal foods (along with saturated fat) which can increase the body's inflammation levels.

**Arthralgia.** Point in the joints.

**Arthritis.** Inflammation of joints. There are more than 100 types of arthritis.

**Articular cartilage.** Cushioned, watery, highly slick cartilage in the area of the joints at the ends of bones.

**Autoimmune.** A process by which the body's immune system turns on or attacks the body's own tissues. Rheumatoid arthritis is considered an autoimmune disease.

**Bacteria.** Microscopic one-celled organisms.

**Bioflavonoids.** Substances once known as vitamin P and closely related in nature to ascorbic acid. These water-soluble compounds are generally yellow in coloration and found in citrus, rose hips and other plants. Plants richest in bioflavonoids are often most colorful. They are powerful antioxidants and also help to maintain the structure and integrity of the body's collagen.

**Bone marrow.** Soft, vascular tissue in the cavities of bones where blood cells are formed.

**Cartilage.** Firm, white-blue substance at ends of bones. Highly water-dependent. Has no blood vessels. Acts as body's shock absorber.

**Chondrocytes.** The cells in joints that produce the substances that make up cartilage.

**Circulating immune complex.** A globulin of antibodies and antigens with other tissue matter that is formed during some inflammatory and autoimmune diseases, such as rheumatoid arthritis, and may be deposited in the body's tissues, causing intense inflammation.

**Collagen.** Substance making up body's connective tissues. Collagen gives cartilage its "spring." The collagen found in joints is called Collagen type II.

**Corticosteroid.** Powerful steroid medication that reduces inflammation. Complications include damage to heart, bone, immune systems. Inhibits the production of prostaglandins and white blood cells.

**Crepitus.** The crackling sound joints make.

**Cyst.** Sac of fluid that forms in bone as cartilage is worn away.

**Duodenal ulcer.** A sore in the mucous membranes located in the first portion of the small intestine.

**Fascia.** A band or sheath of connective tissue covering, supporting or connecting the muscles or internal organs of the body.

**Free radical.** Substance or molecular fragment with one or more unpaired electrons. It is highly reactive, stripping and damaging other cells in a process called oxidation as it searches for an electron match.

**Glucosamine.** An amino sugar occurring in vertebrate tissues including that of marine shells and other small marine creatures from where it is usually harvested.

**Glucosamine sulfate (or sulphate).** A specific form of glucosamine used as an osteoarthritis healing agent.

**Glycosaminoglycans.** A group of polysaccharides that are responsible for water retention in cartilage. Glycosaminoglycans are the building blocks of proteoglycans.

**Gout.** Painful inflammation usually of the big toe, characterized by an excess of uric acid in the blood that leads to crystalline deposits in the small joints.

**Health Maintenance Organization (HMO).** Organization that delivers medical services to preselected care givers at a fixed price on a prepaid basis.

**Herb.** A plant valued for its medicinal properties.

**Histamine.** Derived from the amino acid histidine, histamines are released particularly by damaged mast cells during allergic reactions. They cause dilation and blood vessel permeability and may cause inflammation.

**Isometrics.** A form of exercise in which immovable pressure is applied, such as pressing hands against each other or neck against hand, or pushing into a wall.

**Leukotrienes.** Lipids produced by white blood cells in an immune response to antigens that contribute to allergic asthma and inflammatory reactions.

**Ligament.** Band of strong connective tissue that connects bones and holds organs in place.

**Opioid.** Semisynthetic or synthetic opiumlike substance.

**Osteoarthritis.** The wear-and-tear or biomechanical form of arthritis, as opposed to rheumatoid arthritis, which is an autoimmune disease.

**Osteophytes.** Mineralized outgrowths of bone in damaged cartilage areas.

**Passive movement.** Movement initiated or aided by another person.

**Prostaglandins.** Hormone-like fatty acid substances that influence the body's inflammation levels, temperature, muscular contractions and many other functions. As with cholesterol, there are thought to be "good" prostaglandins and "bad" prostaglandins.

**Protein.** Composed of long chains of amino acids and constituting much of the mass of living organisms.

**Proteoglycans.** Mortar-like substances made from protein and sugar that are the building blocks of cartilage.

**Rheumatoid arthritis.** Autoimmune form of arthritis.

**Slow-acting drug in osteoarthritis.** Specific term applied to glucosamine sulfate by the International League Against Rheumatism.

**Sulfate.** Derived from sulfuric acid and a nutrient for the body's joint matrix and other tissues.

**Synovial fluid.** A clear, viscous, lubricating fluid found in joints.

**Synovial membrane (or synovium).** The soft encapsulating material surrounding the joint that allows nutrients and toxins and other liquids to pass in and out.

**Tendons.** White fibrous cord or band that connects muscles to bones.

**Thromboxane.** Substance formed in blood platelets that causes clotting.

# Resources

*Glucosamine sulfate and other supplements*

Enzymatic Therapy
825 Challenger Drive
Green Bay, WI 54311
(800) 783-2286
Web page: **www.enzy.com.**
*Source of GS-500, the glucosamine sulfate product produced by Rotta Research Laboratories which is proved effective in clinical trials with more than 6,000 patients. Available to the public at health food stores nationwide and to health professionals through the Phytopharmica line. Other products include the Doctor's Choice line of multiple vitamin, mineral and phytochemical daily supplements for men, women and teens; Doctor's Choice antioxidant formula; and a quality St. John's wort supplement called HyperiCalm.™*

## Vitamin E

Carlson Labs
15 West College Drive
Arlington Heights, IL 60004-1985
(800) 323-4141
E-mail: **carlson@carlsonlabs.com.**
*E-Gems are an excellent and naturally sourced form of vitamin E.*

## Combination oral enzyme formula

Marlyn Nutraceuticals/Naturally Vitamins
14851 North Scottsdale Road
Scottsdale, Arizona 85254
(800) 899-4499
Web page: **www.naturallyvitamins.com.**
*Exclusive North American distributor of Wobenzym N, a recommended oral combination enzyme formula widely available in health food stores.*

## Transbuccal vitamins and minerals

Mayor Pharmaceutical Laboratories
2401 South 24th Street
Phoenix, AZ 85036
(800) 582-5273
*For individuals with digestive problems or who cannot swallow capsules, spray vitamins and minerals may help.*

## Rain Forest herbs

Lotus Brands, Inc.
Box 325
Twin Lakes, WI 53181
(800) 824-6396 or (414) 889-8561
*Exclusive distributor of Rainforest Remedies, which are gath-
ered with prayer and care according to ancient Mayan tradition.
Their Flex-Free formula, available at health food stores, employs
traditionally used China root and wild yam root to support joint
function and flexibility.*

## Doctors likely to be familiar with glucosamine sulfate

To locate a health practitioner who is knowledgeable about
glucosamine sulfate and who emphasizes a natural healing program
utilizing concepts reported in this book, contact the following
groups:

American Academy of Anti-aging Medicine
90 South Cascade Avenue,
Colorado Springs, CO 80903
(719) 475-8775
FAX: (719) 475-8748

American Association of Naturopathic Physicians
2366 Eastlake Avenue
Seattle, WA 98102
(206) 323-7610

American Chiropractic Association
1701 Clarendon Boulevard
Arlington, VA 22209
(703) 276-8800

American College of Advancement of Medicine
23121 Verdugo Drive
Laguna Hills, CA 92653
(714) 583-7666

Gladys Taylor McGarey Medical Foundation
7350 East Stretson Drive
Scottsdale, AZ 85251
(602) 946-4544
FAX: (602) 946-6902
Web site: **www.primenet.com~gtmmfihc**
E-mail: **gtmmfihc@primenet.com.**
*Dedicated to bringing the honored traditions of healing to individuals and health care professionals by embracing a holistic philosophy. Publishes* HealthLinks. *A resource center for physicians and patients seeking information and referrals.*

## Organizations dedicated to dealing with arthritis and pain

**American Academy of Medical Acupuncture**
5820 Wilshire Boulevard
Los Angeles, CA
(213) 937-5514

**American Academy of Orthopedic Medicine**
90 South Cascade Avenue
Colorado Springs, CO 80903
(800) 992-2063

**American Academy of Pain Management**
13947 Mono Way #A
Sonora, CA 95370
(209) 533-9750

**American Academy of Pain Medicine, American Chronic Pain Association, American Chronic Pain Outreach Association, Inc.**
4700 West Lake Avenue
Glenview, IL
(847) 375-4731

**American Pain Society**
5700 Old Orchard Tree Road
Skokie, IL
(708) 966-5595

**Arizona Pain Institute**
2601 East Roosevelt
Phoenix, AZ 85008
(800) 559-PAIN

**Arthritis Foundation**
1330 West Peachtree
Atlanta, GA 30309
(404) 872-7100 or (800) 283-7800
Website: **www.arthritis.org.** or **help@arthritis.org**

**International Pain Foundation**
909 Northeast 43rd Street
Seattle, WA 98105
(206) 547-2157

## *Testing for allergic and immune forms of arthritis*

Immuno Labs, Inc.
1620 West Oakland Park Boulevard
Fort Lauderdale, FL 33311
(800) 231-9197

## *Prolotherapy information*

Megan Shields, M.D., one of the coauthors of this book, has a
website on prolotherapy which she employs as a healing modality
at her health center. You can learn much more about this important
healing pathway at her website: **www.prolotherapy.com.**

## *Nutrient testing*

Metametrix
(800) 221-4640
*Amino acid and fatty acid test.*

Spectracell Labs
(800) 227-5227
*B vitamin tests.*

Doctor's Data
(800) 323-2784
*Mineral testing.*

Pantox
(888) 726-8698
*Antioxidant and coenzyme Q10 test.*

## The Doctors' Prescription for Healthy Living

*The authors of this book publish or contribute to* The Doctors' Prescription for Healthy Living, *a newsletter dedicated to informing consumers about the safe brands of household cleaning products, cosmetics, personal care products, foods and nutritional supplements that they shop for on a daily basis. The newsletter makes brand name recommendations after carefully researching available products and also teaches consumers about medically validated pathways of natural healing for conditions such as depression, enlarged prostate, menopausal symptoms, high blood pressure and cholesterol, diabetes, obesity and other common health problems. $19.95 for 12 issues or $34.95 for 24 issues. Send your check or money order to Freedom Press, 1801 Chart Trail, Topanga, CA 90290.*

## To support health freedom

Association of American Physicians and Surgeons, Inc.
1601 North Tucson Boulevard
Tucson, AZ 85716
(800) 635-1196
FAX: (520) 326-3529

*An organization dedicated to preserving the free practice of medicine and the autonomy of physicians. If you're going to battle Medicare or HMOs, this is the group you want to have behind you.*

Arizona Board of Homeopathic Medical Examiners
1400 West Washington
Phoenix, AZ 85007
(602) 543-3095
FAX: (602) 543-3093

Citizens for Health
P.O. Box 2260
Boulder, CO 80306
(303) 417-0772
FAX: (303) 417-9378
*National grass roots health freedom group dedicated to advancing consumer power. Memberships are $15 annually and help protect to your health freedoms including access to medical treatments of your choice. Co-author David Steinman is chairman.*

U.S. Office of Alternative Medicine
National Institutes of Health
9000 Rockville Pike
Bethesda, MD 20892
(301) 402-2466
*Excellent source for information on alternative medical therapies and funding of research into alternative medicine.*

# References

1 Percival, M. *Healthy Answers*, Fall 1997: 4.
2 Lequesne, M., et al. "Guidelines for testing slow-acting drugs in osteoarthritis." *Journal of Rheumatology*, 1994; 21: 65–73.
3 "Anti-Inflammatory Drug Wins Approval from FDA." *The Wall Street Journal*. July 7, 1997: B7.
4 McIlwain, H.H. & Fulghum Bruce, D. *Stop Osteoarthritis Now!* New York, NY: Simon & Schuster, 1996, p. 180.
5 The Burton Goldberg Group. *Alternative Medicine: The Definitive Guide*. Puyallup, WA: Future Medicine Publishing, Inc., p. 531.
6 Clayman, C. [medical editor]. *The American Medical Association Family Medical Guide*. New York, NY: Random House: 1994, p. 589.
7 Cimmino M.A. "Recognition and management of bacterial arthritis." *Drugs*, 1997 July, 54(1):50–60.
8 Murray, M.T. & Pizzorno, J.E. *Encyclopedia of Natural Medicine*, Rocklin, CA: Prima Publishing, 1991.
9 Clayman [medical editor]. *The AMA Family Medical Guide*, p. 588.
10 O'Brien, M.E. & Hoel, D. "Overpowering pain. A serious problem comes out of the closet." *Postgraduate Medicine*, October 1997: 4–10.
11 *The PDR Family Guide to Prescription Drugs*. Montvale, NJ: Medical Economics, 1995, p. 831.
12 *The Use of Opioids for the Treatment of Chronic Pain*. A consensus

statement from the American Academy of Pain Medicine and American Pain Society, 1997. Call 1-847-375-4731 to obtain the report.

13 Crolle, G. & D'Este, E. "Glucosamine sulfate for the management of arthrosis: a controlled clinical investigation." *Current Medical Research and Opinion*, 1980; 7(2): 104–109.

14 Pujalte, J.M., et al. "Double-blind clinical evaluation of oral glucosamine sulphate in the basic treatment of osteoarthrosis." *Current Medical Research and Opinion*, 1980; 7(2): 110–114.

15 Newman, N.M. & Ling, R.S.M. "Acetabular bone destruction related to nonsteroidal anti-inflammatory drugs." *Lancet*, 1985; ii: 11–13.

16 Solomon, L. "Drug-induced arthropathy and necrosis of the femoral head." *Journal of Bone and Joint Surgery*, 1973; 55B: 246–251.

17 Ronningen, H. & Langeland, N. "Indomethacin treatment in osteoarthritis of the hip joint." *Acta Orthop Scand*, 1979; 50: 169–174.

18 Müller-Faßender, H., et al. "Glucosamine sulfate compared to ibuprofen in osteoarthritis of the knee." *Osteoarthritis and Cartilage*, 1994; 2: 61–69.

19 Spencer-Green, G. "Drug treatment of arthritis. Update on conventional and less conventional methods." *Postgraduate Medicine*, 1993; 93(7): 129–140.

20 Piperno, M., et al. "Glucosamine sulfate modulates *in vitro* certain dysregulated functions of human osteoarthritis chondrocytes." Manuscript submitted to *Osteoarthritis and Cartilage* for publication.

21 Krajickova, J. & Macek, J. "Urinary proteoglycan degradation production excretion in patients with rheumatoid arthritis and osteoarthritis." *Annals of the Rheumatic Diseases*, 1988: 468–471.

22 Vidal y Plana, R.R., et al. "Articular cartilage pharmacology: I. *In vitro* studies on glucosamine and nonsteroidal antiinflammatory drugs." *Pharmacological Research Communications*, 1978; 10(6): 557–569.

23 Setnikar, R., et al. "Pharmacokinetics of glucosamine in man." *Drug Research*, 1993; 43(II), Nr. 10: 1109–1113.

24 Setnikar, R., et al. "Absorption, distribution and excretion of

radioactivity after a single intravenous or oral administration of [$^{14}$C]-glucosamine to the rat." *Pharmatherapeutica*, 1984; 3: 538–550.

25  Dziewiatkoswski, D.D. *J.Biol. Chem.*, 1951; 189: 187.

26  Kim, J.J., Cornard, H.E.J. *Biol. Chem.*, 1974; 249: 3091.

27  Thompson, R.C., Jr. & Oeogema, T.R., Jr. "Metabolic activity of articular cartilage in osteoarthritis. An *in vitro* study." *Journal of Bone and Joint Surgery*, 1979; 61(3): 407–416.

28  Bucci, L. *Pain Free*, Lenexa, KS: Wilie International, Inc.

29  Crolle, G. & D'Este, E. "Glucosamine sulfate for the management of arthrosis: a controlled clinical investigation." *Current Medical Research and Opinion*, 1980; 7(2): 104–114.

30  Rovati, L.C. "The practical clinical development of a selective drug for osteoarthritis: glucosamine sulfate." Presented at EULAR '96, Madrid, October 7–10, 1996.

31  Drovani, A., et al. "Therapeutic activity of oral glucosamine sulfate in osteoarthrosis: A placebo-controlled double-blind investigation." *Clinical Therapeutics*, 1980; 3(4): 260–272.

32  D'Ambrosio, E., et al. "Glucosamine sulphate: a controlled clinical investigation in arthrosis." *Pharmatherapeutica*, 1981; 2(8): 504–508.

33  Lopes Vaz, A. "Double-blind clinical evaluation of the relative efficacy of ibuprofen and glucosamine sulphate in the management of osteoarthritis of the knee in outpatients." *Current Medical Research and Opinion*, 1982; 8: 145–149.

34  Tapadinhas, M.J., et al. "Oral glucosamine sulphate in the management of arthrosis: report on a multicentre open investigation in Portugal." *Pharmatherapeutica*, 1982; 3(3): 157–167.

35  Rovati, L.C. "Clinical research in osteoarthritis: design and results of short-term and long-term trials with disease-modifying drugs." *International Journal of Tissue Reactions*, 1992; 14(5): 243–251.

36  Noack, W., et al. "Glucosamine sulfate in oseoarthritis of the knee." *Osteoarthritis and Cartilage*, 1994; 2: 51–59.

37  Rovati, L.C., et al. "A large, randomized, placebo-controlled, double-blind study of glucosamine sulfate vs. piroxicam and vs. their association, on the kinetics of the symptomatic effect in knee osteoarthritis." *Osteoarthritis and Cartilage*, 2 (suppl. 1): 56, 1994.

38 Müller-Faßender, H., et al. "Glucosamine sulfate compared to ibuprofen." *Osteoarthritis and Cartilage* 1994; 2: 61–69.

39 Giordano, N., et al. "The efficacy and safety of glucosamine sulfate in the treatment of gonarthritis." *Clinica Terapeutica*, 1996; 147(3): 99–105.

40 Setnikar, I., et al. "Antiarthritic effects of glucosamine sulfate studied in animal models." *Arzneimittel-Forschung*, 1991; 41(5): 542–545.

41 McCarty, M.F. "The neglect of glucosamine as a treatment for osteoarthritis—a personal perspective." *Medical Hypotheses*, 1994; 42(5): 323–327.

42 Murray & Pizzorno. *Encyclopedia of Natural Medicine*, pp. 493–494.

43 Panush, R.S. "Food-induced (allergic) arthritis: inflammatory arthritis exacerbated by milk." *Arthritis and Rheumatism*, 1986; 29(2): 220–225.

44 Darlington, L.G., et al. "Placebo-controlled, blind study of dietary manipulation therapy in rheumatoid arthritis." *Lancet*, February 1, 1986: 236–238.

45 Ratner, D., et al. "Juvenile rheumatoid arthritis and milk allergy." *Journal of the Royal Society of Medicine*, 1985; 78(5): 410–413.

46 Panush, R.S. "Food-induced ('allergic') arthritis: inflammatory synovitis in rabbits." *The Journal of Rheumtology*, 1990; 17: 285–290.

47 Kjeldsen-Kragh, J. "Controlled trial of fasting and one-year vegetarian diet in rheumatoid arthritis." *Lancet*, 1991; 338(8772): 899–902.

48 Williams, R. "Rheumatoid arthritis and food: a case study." *British Medical Journal*, 1981; 283: 563.

49 Williams, R. Cited in Carper, J. *Food—Your Miracle Medicine*. HarperCollins Publishers, 1993, pp. 372–373.

50 Carper, J. *Food—Your Miracle Medicine*, pp. 373–374.

51 Darlington, L.G. "Dietary therapy for arthritis." *Nutrition and Rheumatic Diseases*, 1991; 17(2): 273–285.

52 Houston, L. & Ursell, A. "Dietary change in arthritis." *The Practitioner*, June 1994; 238: 443–448.

53 Ursell, A. *The Practitioner*, 238: 284–288.

54 Shapiro, J.A., et al. "Diet and rheumatoid arthritis in women: a possible protective effect of fish consumption." *Epidemiology*, 1996 May, 7(3):256–63.

55 Carper. *Food—Your Miracle Medicine*, pp. 380–381.

56 Corman, L.C. "The role of diet in animal models of systemic lupus erythematosus: possible implications for human lupus." *Seminars in Arthritis and Rheumatism*, 1985; 15(1): 61–69.

57 Robinson, D.R., et al. "The protective effect of dietary fish oil on murine lupus." *Prostaglandins*, 1985; 30(1): 51–75.

58 Kelley, V.E., et al. "A fish oil diet rich in eicosapentaenoic acid reduces cyclooxygenase metabolites, and suppresses lupus in MRL-lpr mice." *Journal of Immunity*, 1985; 134(3): 1914–1919.

59 "Prevalence of leisure-time physical activity among persons with arthritis and other rheumatic conditions—United States, 1990–1991." *Mmwr. Morbidity and Mortality Weekly Report*, 1997 May 9, 46(18): 389–93.

60 Ettinger W.H., Jr., & Afable, R.F. "Physical disability from knee osteoarthritis: the role of exercise as an intervention." *Medicine and Science in Sports and Exercise*, 1994; 26(12): 1435–1440.

61 Ytterberg, S.R., et al. "Exercise for arthritis." *Baillieres Clinical Rheumatology*, 1994; 8(1): 161–189.

62 Fransen M,. et al. "A revised group exercise program for osteoarthritis of the knee." *Physiother. Res. Int.*, 1997; 2(1): 30–41.

63 Borjesson M., et al. "Physiotherapy in knee osteoarthrosis: effect on pain and walking." *Physiother. Res. Int.*, 1996; 1(2): 89–97.

64 Komatireddy G.R., et al. "Efficacy of low-load resistive muscle training in patients with rheumatoid arthritis functional class II and III." *Journal of Rheumatology*, 1997; 24(8): 1531–1539.

65 Neuberger G.B., et al. "Effects of exercise on fatigue, aerobic fitness, and disease activity measures in persons with rheumatoid arthritis." *Research in Nursing and Health*, 1997; 20(3): 195–204.

66 Noreau L., et al. "Dance-based exercise program in rheumatoid arthritis. Feasibility in individuals with American College of Rheumatology functional class III disease." *American Journal of Physical Medicine and Rehabilitation*, 1997; 76(2): 109–113.

67 Melton-Rogers S., et al. "Cardiorespiratory responses of patients

with rheumatoid arthritis during bicycle riding and running in water." *Physical Therapy*, 1996; 76(10): 1058–1065.

68  Lyngberg K.K., et al. "Elderly rheumatoid arthritis patients on steroid treatment tolerate physical training without an increase in disease activity." *Archives of Physical Medicine and Rehabilitation*, 1994; 75(11): 1189–1195.

69  Hakkinen A., et al. "Effects of strength training on neuromuscular function and disease activity in patients with recent-onset inflammatory arthritis." *Scandinavian Journal of Rheumatology*, 1994; 23(5): 237–242.

70  Young, S. "Healthy bones at 20, 30, 40, 50." *Glamour*, January 1993: 38.

71  United Press International. "Exercise, estrogen benefit older women." Not dated.

72  Helliwell, M., et al. *Annals Rheum. Dis.*, 1984; 43: 386–390.

73  "Building immunity. What can help?" *Nutrition Action Health Letter*, September 1997: 1, 4–7.

74  Tappel, A.L. *Free Radical Biology & Medicine*, 1996; 20: 165–173.

75  Kremer, J.M. "Severe rheumatoid arthritis: current options in drug therapy." *Geriatrics*, 1990; 45(12): 43–48.

76  Lau C.S., et al. "Effects of fish oil supplementation on nonsteroidal anti-inflammatory drug requirement in patients with mild rheumatoid arthritis—a double-blind, placebo-controlled study. *British Journal of Rheumatology*, 1993; 32(11): 982–989.

77  Murray, M. *Encyclopedia of Nutritional Supplements*. Rocklin, CA: Prima Publishing, 1996, p. 262.

78  Murray, M., *ibid.*, p. 263.

79  Granato, H. "Prop 65 activists target fish oil." *Natural Foods Merchandiser*, 1997; 18(11): 18.

80  Barton-Wright, E.C. & Elliott, W.A. "The pantothenic acid metabolism of rheumatoid arthritis." *Lancet*, 1963; 2: 862–863.

81  Nelson, M.N., et al. *Proceedings of the Society for Experimental Biology*, 1950; 73: 31.

82  "A report from the General Practitioner Research Group." *Practitioner*, 1980; 224: 208–211.

83  Bates, C.J. "Proline and hydroxyproline excretion and vitamin C status in elderly human subjects." *Clinical Science and Molecular Medicine*, 1977; 52: 535–543.

84 Davis, R.H., et al. "Vitamin C influence on localized adjuvant arthritis." *Journal of the American Podiatric Medical Association*, 1990; 80(8): 414–418.

85 Kheir, Eldin, A.A., et al. "Effect of vitamin C administration in modulating some biochemical changes in arthritic rats." *Pharmacological Research*, 1992; 26(4): 1043–1066.

86 Tarayre, J.P., et al. "Advantages of a combination of proteolytic enzymes, flavonoids and ascorbic acid in comparison with nonsteroid anti-inflammatory agents." *Arzneim-Forsch*, 1977; 27(I): 1144–1149.

87 Machtey, I. & Ouaknine, L. "Tocopherol in osteoarthritis: a controlled pilot study." *Journal of the American Geriatric Society*, 1978; 26: 328.

88 Murray, & Pizzorno. *Encyclopedia of Natural Medicine*, p. 450.

89 Munthe, E. & Aseth, E. "Treatment of rheumatoid arthritis with selenium and vitamin E." *Scandinavian Journal of Rheumatology*, 1984; 53 (suppl.): 103.

90 Panganamala, R.V. & Cornwell, D.G. "The effects of vitamin E on arachidonic acid metabolism." *Annals of the New York Academy of Sciences*, 1982; 393: 376–391.

91 Murray. *Encyclopedia of Nutritional Supplements*, p. 171.

92 Murray & Pizzorno. *Encyclopedia of Natural Medicine*, p. 495.

93 Fernandez-Madrid, F., et al. "Effect of zinc deficiency on collagen metabolism." *Proceedings of the Forty-fourth Annual Meeting*, 78(5): 853.

94 Marcolongo, R., et al. "Double-blind multicentre study of the activity of S-adenosyl-methionine in hip osteoarthritis." *Current Therapeutic Research*, 1985; 37: 82–94.

95 Murray. *Encyclopedia of Nutritional Supplements*, p. 373.

96 Steffen, C., et al. "Enzymtherapie im vergleich mit immunkomplexbestimmungen bei chronischer polyarthritis." *Zeitschr. f. Rheumatologie*, 1985; 44: 51.

97 Streichhan, P., et al. "Resorption partikulärer und makromolekularer Darminhaltsstoffe." *Nature-und Ganzheitsmedizin*, 1988; 1: 90.

98 Miehlke, K. "Enzymtherapie bei rheumatoider arthritis." *Nature-und Ganzheitsmedizin*, 1988; 1:108.

99 Heidland, A., et al. "Renal fibrosis: role of impaired proteolysis and potential therapeutic strategies." *Kidney International*, 1997; 52 (suppl. 62). Paper in press at time of publication; page numbers not available.

100 Carper, J., *Food—Your Miracle Medicine*, p. 487.

101 Carper, J., *ibid.*, p. 383.

102 Cohen, A. & Goldman, J. "Bromelain therapy in rheumatoid arthritis." *Pennsylvania Medical Journal*, 1964; 67: 27–30.

103 Isaka, K. "Gastrointestinal absorption and anti-inflammatory effect of bromelain." *Journal of Japanese Pharmacology*, 1972; 22: 519–534.

104 Vane, J. "The evolution of nonsteroidal anti-inflammatory drugs and their mechanisms of action." *Drugs*, 1987; 33 (Suppl. 1): 18–27.

105 Akamatsu, H., et al. "Mechanism of anti-inflammatory action of glycyrrhizin: effect on neutrophil functions including reactive oxygen species generation." *Planta Medica*, 1991; 57: pp. 119–121.

106 Passwater, R.A. & Kandaswami, C. *Pycnogenol: The Super "Protector" Nutrient*. New Canaan, CT: Keats Publishing, 1994, pp. 94–95.

107 Arvigo, R. & Balick, M.J. *Rainforest Remedies: One Hundred Healing Herbs of Belize*. Twin Lakes, WI: Lotus Press, 1993, pp. 44–45, 194–195.

108 Baici, A., et al. "Analysis of gluycosaminoglycans in human serum after oral administration of chondroitin sulfate." *Rheumatology International*, 1992; 12: 81–88.

109 Prudden, J.F. & Balassa, L.L. "The biological activity of bovine cartilage preparations." *Seminars on Arthritis and Rheumatism*, 1974; 3(4): 287.

110 Kerzberg, E.M., et al. "Combination of glycosaminoglycans and acetylsalicylic acid in knee osteoarthritis." *Scandinavian Journal of Rheumatology*, 1987; 16: 377–380.

111 Rovetta, G. "Galactosaminoglycuronoglycan sulfate (matrix) in therapy of tibiofibular osteoarthritis of the knee." *Drugs in Experimental and Clinical Research*, 1991; 18(1): 53–57.

112 Olivero, U. "Effects of the treatment with matrix on elderly people

with chronic articular degeneration." *Drugs in Experimental and Clinical Research*, 1991; 17(1).

113 Mazières, B., et al. "Le chondroitin sulfate dayns le traitement de la gonarthrose et de la coxarthrose." *Rev. Rheum. Mal Ostéoartic*, 1992; 59(7–8): 466–472.

114 Pipitone, V.R. "Chondroprotection with chondroitin sulfate." *Drugs in Experimental and Clinical Research*, 1991; 17(1): 3–7.

115 Morreale P., et al. "Comparison of the anti-inflammatory efficacy of chondroitin sulfate and diclofenac sodium in patients with knee osteoarthritis." *Journal of Rheumatology*, 1996 Aug, 23(8):1385–1391.

116 Theodosakis, J., et al. *The Arthritis Cure*. New York: St. Martin's Press, 1997, p. xvi.

117 Sahelian, R. *Glucosamine: Nature's Arthritis Remedy*. Marina del Rey, CA: Longevity Research Center, 1997, p. 24.

118 Shute, N. "Aching for an arthritis cure." *U.S. News & World Report*, Feb. 10, 1997.

119 Pelletier, K. *Mind as Healer, Mind as Slayer*. New York, NY: Dell Publishing Co., Inc., 1977, p. 6.

120 Moos, R.H. & Solomon, G.F. "Psychologic comparisons between women with rheumatoid arthritis and their nonarthritic sisters." *Psychosomatic Medicine*, 1965; 2: 150.

121 Solomon, G.F. "Emotions, stress, the central nervous system, and immunity." *Annals of the New York Academy of Sciences*, 1969; 164(2): 335–343.

122 Sahelian, R. "Spotlight shines on St. John's wort." *Whole Foods*, September 1997: 54, 56.

# Index

# The Authors

Between them, these three outstanding physicians have helped thousands of arthritis patients over the years regain their health using the program described in *Arthritis: The Doctors' Cure*.

**Michael W. Loes, M.D., M.D.(H.)** is the director of the Arizona Pain Institute, a division of the University of Arizona's Integrative Program in anesthesiology. He is board certified in internal medicine with subspecialty board certifications in pain medicine and management, addictionology, acupuncture, clinical hypnosis and homeopathy. He is an assistant professor at the University of Arizona Health Science Center, Tucson, and a faculty consultant to the Mayo Clinic's Scottsdale Pain Center.

**Megan Shields, M.D.** has been practicing medicine for more than 20 years. She has won numerous awards for her medical skills, including the Mead Johnson Award for graduate education in family practice and the Golden Apple Award for outstanding teaching at the Long Beach Memoral Medical Center Family Practice Residency Program. A diplomate of the American Board of Family Practice, Dr. Shields has specialized in family practice with an emphasis on natural approaches to healing. She is a member of the science advisory board for the Foundation of Advancements in Science and Education.

**Gary Wikholm, M.D.** is a board-certified specialist in family medicine and a specialist in emergency medicine and obstetrics. He is a qualified medical evaluator in occupational medicine for the state of California and clinical instructor in the Family Medicine Glendale-Adventist Family Practice Residency Program, which is part of Loma Linda University. He is also a clinical instructor in emergency medicine for the Ventura County Medical Center.

**David Steinman** is author or coauthor of *Diet for a Poisoned Planet*, *The Safe Shopper's Bible*, *Living Healthy in a Toxic World*, and *The Breast Cancer Prevention Program*. He is chairman of Citizens for Health, served two years on a committee of the National Academy of Sciences where he coauthored *Seafood Safety.* Publisher of *The Doctors' Prescription for Healthy Living,* Steinman is a member of the teaching faculty at National University and has won awards from the California Newspaper Publishers' Association, Sierra Club and Society of Journalists' *Best of the West.*